Basic EKG Facts

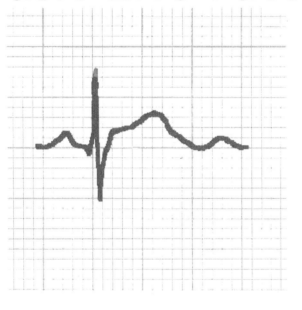

James B. Martin, RN

© Copyright 2004 James B. Martin. All rights reserved.

No part of this publication may be reproduced, stored in a retrieval system, or transmitted, in any form or by any means, electronic, mechanical, photocopying, recording, or otherwise, without the written prior permission of the author.

Note for Librarians: a cataloguing record for this book that includes Dewey Classification and US Library of Congress numbers is available from the National Library of Canada. The complete cataloguing record can be obtained from the National Library's online database at: www.nlc-bnc.ca/amicus/index-e.html
ISBN 1-4120-1710-6

TRAFFORD

This book was published on-demand in cooperation with Trafford Publishing.
On-demand publishing is a unique process and service of making a book available for retail sale to the public taking advantage of on-demand manufacturing and Internet marketing. On-demand publishing includes promotions, retail sales, manufacturing, order fulfilment, accounting and collecting royalties on behalf of the author.

Suite 6E, 2333 Government St., Victoria, B.C. V8T 4P4, CANADA
Phone   250-383-6864   Toll-free 1-888-232-4444 (Canada & US)
Fax   250-383-6804   E-mail   sales@trafford.com
Web site www.trafford.com   TRAFFORD PUBLISHING IS A DIVISION OF TRAFFORD HOLDINGS LTD.
Trafford Catalogue #03-2087   www.trafford.com/robots/03-2087.html
10   9   8   7   6   5   4   3   2   1

To my wife, Beth,
for her encouragement and support,

And

To my sons, Jeremy and Jared,
for the artwork used in this book.

With

A special "Thank You" to all of my co-workers
who encouraged me throughout the writing of this book.

Basic EKG Facts
Table of Contents

Introduction..7

Chapter One..11

Down the Correct Path
    Electrical Anatomy of the Heart

Chapter Two..21

Wires, Wires Everywhere
    Lead Placement
    Electrode Placement Chart

Chapter Three..33

Making Waves

    The Paper
    The Waves

Chapter Four..55

From the Top...Atrial Rhythms
    Sinus Rhythm
    Sinus Bradycardia
    Sinus Tachycardia
    Supraventricular Tachycardia
    Sinus Arrhythmia
    Sinus Arrest
    Sinus Block
    Sick Sinus Syndrome
    Premature Atrial Contractions
    Wandering Atrial Pacemaker
    Atrial Tachycardia
    Multifocal Atrial Tachycardia

Atrial Fibrillation
Atrial Flutter

Chapter Five..89

In the Middle...Junctional Rhythms
> *Junctional Rhythm*
> *Premature Junctional Complexes*
> *Accelerated Junctional Rhythm*
>
> *Junctional Tachycardia*

Chapter Six...97

From the Bottom...Ventricular Rhythms
> *Premature Ventricular Complexes*
> *Ventricular Tachycardia*
> *Torsades de Pointes*
> *Wolfe Parkinson White Syndrome*
> *Aberrant Ventricular Conduction*
> *Ventricular Fibrillation*
> *Accelerated Idioventricular Rhythm*
>
> *Asystole*
>
> *Agonal Rhythm*

Chapter Seven..123

Traffic Delays...Blocks
> *First Degree Block*
> *Second Degree Block Mobitz I*
> *Second Degree Mobitz II*
> *Third Degree Block*
> *Bundle Branch Blocks*

Chapter Eight...139

A Little Help...Pacemakers
> *Permanent*
> *Temporary*

Chapter Nine..153

Odds and Ends...Evens and Middles
    Ischemia and Infarction
    Evolution of an MI
    Axis Determination
    Atrial Enlargement
    Ventricular Hypertrophy
    Common Drug Effects
    Infarction Locator Template

Introduction

If one were to look at a timeline of medical history, events and discoveries would be spaced rather far apart at the beginning and extremely close together as today's date approached. Much of early medicine was based on philosophy rather than biological principal, and it wasn't until Hypocrites distinguished a difference between the two that "modern" medicine began to evolve.

Early cave drawings depict man and animals with hearts at the center of their bodies. The ancient Egyptians are credited with the discovery of the pulse and it's relationship to the circulation of blood, and as early as 600 B.C. the Greeks had distinguished between arteries and veins, and had reasoned that the brain, not the heart, was the center of sensation.

Medicine moved quite slowly into and through the Renaissance period with aseptic techniques, the use of anesthetics and advancements in the study of anatomy being the most noted achievements.

The 17th century brought us advances in physiology, gross pathology, and the clinical study of disease with inventions such as the microscope; while the 18th century brought serious doubt that the science was advancing at all. It did include advances however, such as the development and discoveries of the harnessing of electricity and it's effects on animal tissues. In 1678 frog's legs were found to respond to the passage of an electrical current through the tissues, and in 1775 chickens were rendered lifeless "with a single shock to the head, and then shocked back to life using another shock to the thorax."

Narrowing now to the electrical advances, development moved somewhat faster during the 19th century; techniques became more refined, and inventions of various pieces of equipment advanced discoveries forward. The galvanometer was invented in 1880. It consisted of a magnetized needle, which moved when an electrical current would flow through a surrounding wire coil. The tracings were recorded on a paper moving at a fixed speed. In 1887 Augustus D. Waller published the first human EKG, and in 1893 Willem Einthoven introduced the term electrocardiogram to the Dutch Medical Association.

A timeline of the 20th century would include these highlights:

1902-Einthoven publishes the first human EKG using a string galvanometer, which weighs 600 pounds

1908- The University of Edinburgh purchases the first string galvanometer for clinical use

1909- EKG changes are noted during an angina attack

1920- EKG changes are noted during an acute myocardial infarction

1924- Einthoven wins the Nobel Prize

1926- An Australian physician, who wished to remain unknown because of ethical considerations at the time, resuscitates a newborn using a device later to be called a pacemaker.

1928- the first portable EKG machine, weighing 50 pounds and powered by a car battery, is introduced.

1931- a pacemaker small enough to fit into a doctor's bag (and powered by a hand crank) is introduced.

1942- The 12 lead EKG is introduced.

1947- the first successful defibrillation of a human, a 14-year-old boy, is recorded.

1949- the first monitor capable of sending a continuous signal is introduced. It was carried in a backpack and weighed 75 pounds.

1950- the first pacemaker is invented. It used vacuum tubes and was powered by 60-cycle household current.

1960- R on T significance was discovered.

1968- Marriott introduces the use of MCL1 for continuous EKG monitoring

Now, as we move into the 21st century, we see advances being made in the treatment and/or prevention of arrhythmias more so, than the discovery of previously unknown rhythms. Advances are being made in the medications used for treatment as well as in the equipment available. Drugs are being developed, modified, and evaluated, all in the path to better patient care and safety. Numerous advances have been made in the area of equipment available for patient testing and treatment. Microelectronics have made equipment easier to use, allowed each piece of equipment to do more and considerably reduced the size and weight of each piece. In the first part of the twentieth century a pacemaker was powered by a hand crank, and was considered an advancement because it was small enough "to fit in a doctor's bag." Today pacemakers and defibrillators are no larger or heavier than a few coins stacked together, are implanted into the patient, have batteries that last for years, are computer programmed, can monitor and record events for future review, and have minimal, if any, inconvenience to the patient's lifestyle.

The focus of this book is on the identification and causes of the most common cardiac rhythms. It is not intended to be all-inclusive, because as I write, and re-write this, I am still learning. A brief list of common treatment options is given with each rhythm. This list is neither complete nor specific, as identification, rather than treatment is the goal of this book. Treatment should be based upon correlation of clinical findings along with EKG interpretation rather that a standard "one size fits all" approach, as each patient and situation is individual and should be addressed as such.

It is my hope that this book will serve as a resource of information to assist you in building a solid base of knowledge upon which to grow.

Chapter One

Down the Correct Path

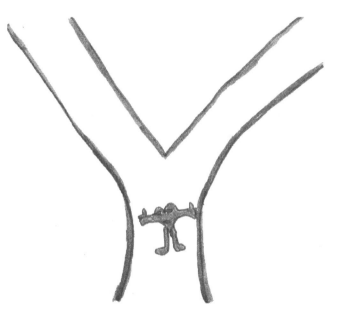

Electrical Anatomy of The Heart

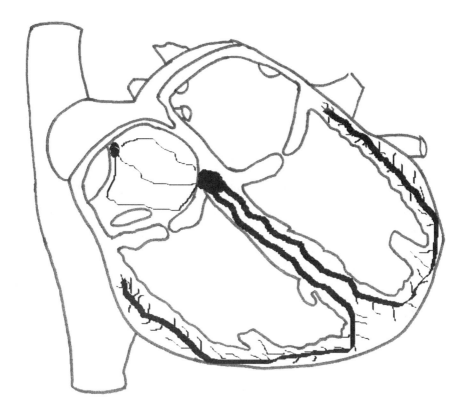

Adequate pumping action of the heart is dependant upon rhythmic contraction of the atria and ventricles, as well as proper functioning of the valves. Each mechanical action is triggered by a chemical action and reaction called action potential. These potentials are triggered by one of several rhythmic pacemaker sites within the heart itself. The action is conducted rapidly throughout the organ to produce a coordinated reaction.

The Sinus Node

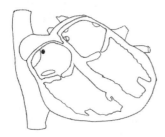

The sinus node is the primary pacemaker of the heart. It is a collection of specialized cardiac cells measuring approximately 15x5x2 mm located in the right atrium near the entrance of the superior vena cava. P cells within the sinus node are thought to be the source of impulse formation. Sympathetic and parasympathetic nerve fibers in the region may increase or decrease impulse formation to vary the heart rate. Internodal tracts carry the impulse through the atria to the atrioventricular node. It takes about 150 milliseconds for the impulse to travel throughout the atria and reach the AV node.

The Internodal Pathways

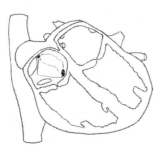

The Internodal pathways are not actual physical pathways, but rather preferred pathways through the atria that conduct the electrical impulse from the SA node to the AV node. Studies indicate there is no morphological difference between the conductive cells and the surrounding cells of the atria, but the geometry of the cells making up the atrial septum and right atrial free wall may represent three potential internodal pathways.

The Atrioventricular Node

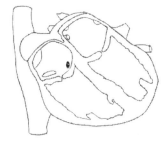

The AV node is normally the only conducting bridge between the atria and ventricles. It is located at the bottom of the right atrium and measures approximately 6x4x1.5 mm. The primary function of the AV node is to momentarily hold the electrical impulse, then release it to allow for smooth coordinated action between the atria and ventricles. This 70-80 ms delay is enough to allow blood to flow through the valves into the lower chambers of the heart to cease and the valves to close creating an effective two stage pump. When released, the impulse travels through the ventricular conduction system; which includes the bundle of His, the right and left bundle branches and the Purkinje system. This system spreads the impulse through the muscle cells of the inner walls of the ventricles. This depolarization of the ventricles takes about 80 ms.

The Bundle of His

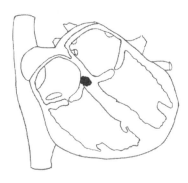

The Bundle of His begins at the distal portion of the AV node and travels through the fibrous body of the ventricular septum. Functioning as the only normal pathway between the atria and ventricles, it is made up of numerous parallel bundles of specialized cardiac muscle cells (Purkinje cells) separated by fibrous tissue, and is insulated by a collagenous sheath. It measures approximately 1 – 2 mm in diameter by 7 – 20 mm in length and forms a cord that divides into the left and right bundle branches.

The Bundle Branches

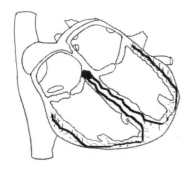

The Bundle Branches, labeled left and right, are a continuation of the Bundle of His. Measuring approximately 1mm in diameter and 50mm in length, they extend down the ventricular septum toward the apex and branch multiple times to form a network of sorts encasing most of the ventricular mass. It takes approximately 40 to 120 milliseconds for an impulse to travel from the AV node throughout the ventricles.

The Pacemakers

Some specialized cells of the heart have the ability to spontaneously generate impulses and function as a type of "back up" pacemaker in the event the normal pacer(s) of the heart are unable to do so. Cells with pacemaker properties are found in the SA node, the AV junction and the Purkinje fibers of the ventricles.

When functioning properly the SA node discharges at a rate of 60-80 times per minute, the AV node around 50 times per minute and the Purkinje system about 40. Firing of the SA node determines the heart rate and the lower pacemakers are reset during each cardiac cycle. Cholinergic stimulation via the vagus nerve results in a slowing of the heart rate while sympathetic stimulation or circulating symptomatic hormones will increase the heart rate.

The Ions

Electrical impulses are caused by chemical changes within the cells of the heart. The membrane surrounding each cell is semi-permeable, that is, certain substances are allowed to pass through, while others are restricted. In the case of the cardiac cells, Potassium (K+) and Sodium (Na) are passed and or restricted. In the resting phase (diastole) the concentration of potassium is high and that of sodium is low within the cell. The cell is negatively charged in relation to the outside. As the cell membrane becomes depolarized (positively charged in relation to the outside), the permeability changes allowing sodium ions to enter the cell. As this happens the sodium concentration within the cell becomes higher than the potassium concentration, and the entire cell is now positively charged resulting the formation of a complex. When this occurs in the atria, a P wave is generated on the EKG. In the ventricles, this action triggers a QRS complex.

Calcium also plays a key role in regulating the contractile process. Depolarization of the cell membrane with its associated inward calcium current triggers the release of additional calcium ions from intracellular stores. The increased concentration of calcium disables an inhibitor protein therefore permitting an action, which leads to a mechanical contraction.

The resting cell has a negative charge when compared to its surroundings.

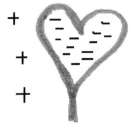

An electrical impulse carries a positive charge into the cell changing its polarity.

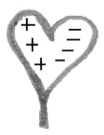

This is called depolarization, which occurs as a contraction.

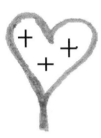

As the electrical impulse leaves the cell, it returns to its resting state, repolarized, awaiting another stimulus.

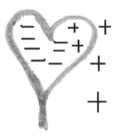

Chapter Two

Wires, Wires, Everywhere

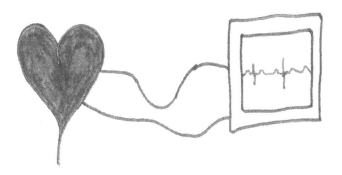

Lead Placement

Proper lead placement and good skin contact are essential to obtaining accurate and consistent EKGs. Good skin contact ensures a clean signal to the electrode, which allows for a smooth tracing. Consistent lead placement allows for proper interpretation as well as ensuring uniformity of future readings.

The arm electrodes are placed on the front of the deltoid muscle for the 12 lead reading or may be placed on the upper portion of the pectoral muscle for continuous, ambulatory monitoring. The arm electrodes may at times be repositioned to allow for pacemaker locations.

The leg electrodes are placed above the ankles for 12 lead views and are relocated to the mid axillary line at or below the umbilicus for continuous, ambulatory monitoring. Electrodes for the limb leads are sometimes placed on the chest wall near the extremity that they represent.

Ten wires, each placed in its own specific location are used to obtain either a twelve or eighteen lead view. To further understand lead placement, the views can be broken down into groups.

Limb leads- Leads I, II, III, aVR, aVL, and aVF- Provide frontal plane views, or side-to-side views. These readings are obtained through the use of the three electrodes attached to the arms and left leg.

LIMB LEADS

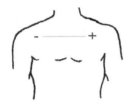

Lead I
R arm NEG
L arm POS

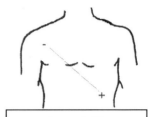

Lead II
R arm NEG
L leg POS

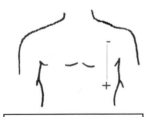

Lead III
L arm NEG
L leg POS

UNIPOLAR LIMBLEADS

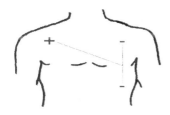

aVR
The positive electrode is placed on the right arm. The left arm and left leg are negative.

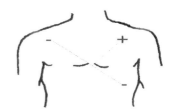

aVL
The positive electrode is placed on the left arm. The right arm and left leg are negative.

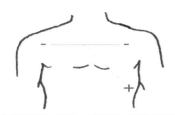

aVF
The positive electrode is placed on the left leg.
The right and left arms are negative.

Precordial leads- Leads V1-V6 – Provide horizontal plane views, or views from the front to the back. These readings are obtained from electrodes attached to the mid chest.

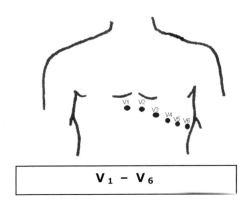

$V_1 - V_6$

Bipolar leads- Leads I, II, and III measure changes in potential between two electrodes:

        Lead I - between both arms

        Lead II – between the right arm and left foot

        Lead III - between the left arm and left foot

Unipolar leads- Leads aVR, aVL, and aVF – are augmented, meaning a current reading is averaged between two limb electrodes and compared to the third. Unipolar leads are best understood imagining an equilateral triangle superimposed over the body with the heart at its center, and it's sides representing the limb leads. This imaginary triangle is known as Einthoven's triangle, named after the Dutch physicist Willem Einthoven, who developed the mathematical equation, which it represents.

        aVR- between the right arm and left arm, left foot combination aVL- between the left arm and right arm, left foot combination

aVF- between the left foot and left art, right arm combination

Right Precordial leads- Leads V_1 - V_2 placed along the right lateral and posterior rib area. These leads give views of the right ventricle, and are used in ST segment monitoring which is useful in the detection of right ventricular injuries and infarctions.

A special marking, a written label or a colored band, identifies each of the chest leads. On many machines these wires are interchangeable. Do not always rely on the markings, rather, follow the lead from its origin and attach it in the appropriate position on the chest.

V_1 - 4th intercostal space at the right sternal border
V_2 - 4th intercostal space at the left sternal border
V_3 - midway between V2 and V4 (this means you cannot just place one lead after the other)
V_4 - 5th intercostal space at the left mid clavicular line
V_5 - midway between V4 and V6
V_6 - 5th intercostal space at the left mid axillary line

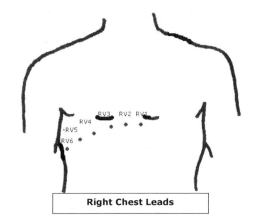

Right Chest Leads

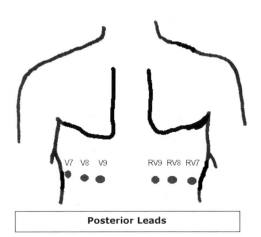

Posterior Leads

INDICATIONS FOR THE USE OF ADDITIONAL PRECORDIAL LEADS:
1. Symptomatic patients presenting with EKGs that are normal or have non-specific changes.
2. Patients with inferior lead changes or reciprocal changes of ST segment depression as seen in a posterior infarction.
    - ♥ ST segment elevation suggestive of an Inferior wall MI (II, III, aVF)
    - ♥ Isolated ST segment elevation in V_1 (or V_2 greater than V_1)
    - ♥ Borderline ST elevation in V_5 & V_6 or in V_1 through V_3
    - ♥ ST depression, or suspicious isolectric segment in V_1 through V_3

ST segment elevation in V_4R through V_6R can resolve in as little as twelve to eighteen hours, so 15 or 18 lead EKGs are most beneficial when obtained as close to the onset of symptoms as possible.

The presence of an anterior wall MI obscures the changes visible in the right precordial leads.

ELECTRODE PLACEMENT		
BIPOLAR LEADS	**POSITIVE**	**NEGATIVE**
I	LEFT ARM	RIGHT ARM
II	LEFT LEG	RIGHT ARM
III	LEFT LEG	LEFT ARM
AUGMENTED LEADS		
aVR	RIGHT ARM	LEFT ARM & LEFT LEG
aVL	LEFT ARM	RIGHT ARM & LEFT LEG
aVF	LEFT LEG	RIGHT ARM & LEFT ARM
PRECORDIAL LEADS	**POSITION**	
V_1	4TH INTERCOSTAL SPACE LEFT - STERNAL BORDER	
V_2	4TH INTERCOSTAL SPACE RIGHT - STERNAL BORDER	
V_3	MIDWAY BETWEEN V2 & V4	
V_4	5TH INTERCOSTAL SPACE MID-CLAVICULAR LINE	
V_5	MIDWAY BETWEEN V4 & V6	
V_6	5TH INTERCOSTAL SPACE MID-AXILLARY LINE	
V_7	LEFT POSTERIOR AXILLARY LINE – STRAIGHT LINE FROM V6	USE V4 ELECTRODE
V_8	LEFT MID SCAPULAR LINE – STRAIGHT LINE FROM V7	USE V5 ELECTRODE
V_9	LEFT PARASPINAL LINE – STRAIGHT LINE FROM V8	USE V6 ELECTRODE

RIGHT CHEST LEADS		
V_1R	4TH INTERCOSTAL SPACE LEFT - STERNAL BORDER	
V_2R	4TH INTERCOSTAL SPACE RIGHT - STERNAL BORDER	
V_3R	MIDWAY BETWEEN V2R & V4R	
V_4R	5TH INTERCOSTAL SPACE RIGHT - MID CLAVICULAR LINE	
V_5R	5TH INTERCOSTAL SPACE RIGHT - BETWEEN V4R & V6R	
V_6R	5TH INTERCOSTAL SPACE RIGHT – MID AXILLARY LINE	

Chapter Three

Making Waves

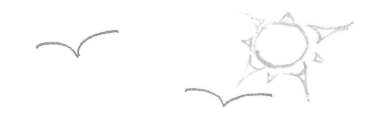

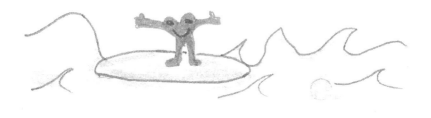

The Paper

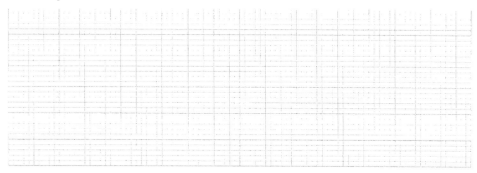

A heat sensitive paper passes a heated stylus at a given speed in order to record EKG tracings onto it. The standard speed is 25 millimeters per second, but for clarification the paper speed can be doubled to 50mm/sec.

The paper is divided in a graph style to allow ease of measurement of the complexes, with each small square on the paper measuring 1mm wide by 1 mm tall. Every fifth line is darkened in both directions, and timing marks appear every fifteen large boxes.

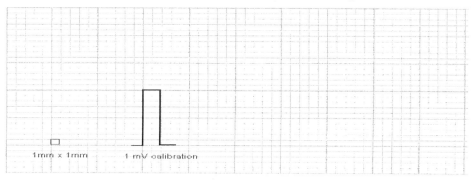

Vertical lines measure the amplitude of the complexes. Ten small boxes (10 mm) represent one millivolt (1mV). The EKG machine should be calibrated so that 1mV equals two large squares. A confirmation of such calibration usually appears at the bottom of the printed EKG.

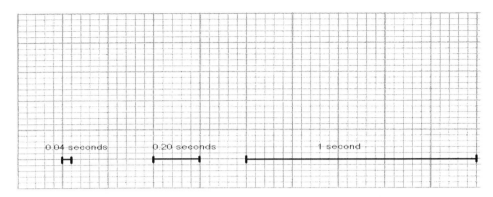

Horizontal lines are used to measure time. Each 1mm box represents 0.04 seconds or 40 milliseconds and five large boxes represent one second when the paper is moving at the standard 25mm/sec speed. If the paper speed is increased to 50mm/sec, the values of each block are halved, thus one small block now represents 0.02 sec, and ten large boxes will pass the stylus in one second. This setting is useful for determining rhythms with fast rates.

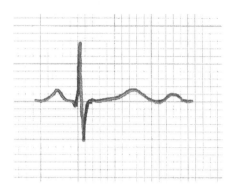

The Waves

The EKG machine transforms the electrical impulses detected by the surface electrodes into a waveform that is printed onto a moving paper. When no electrical activity in detected, a flat line is printed. This line, called the isolectric line, is considered the baseline for the EKG tracing. Electrical activity traveling toward the recording electrode produces an upward or positive waveform, while an impulse traveling away from the electrode will produce a downward or negative waveform. Impulses traveling first in one direction and then in the opposite will produce a waveform that prints both above and below the baseline. This is called a biphasic waveform.

Six major waves, along with various other "points" and complexes, are labeled. The letters P, Q, R, S, T, and U are used to identify them.

The first labels given to the waveforms produced were simply A, B, C, and D. The galvanometer produced sluggish fluctuations and the waveforms could only be seen after tedious calculations were made. In 1891 the galvanometer was improved, electrodes were placed on the right hand and over the apex of the heart, and a complex was recorded with each beat of the heart. Not knowing if these were the same complexes seen in earlier observations, they were labeled P, Q, R, S, and T. These are the first letters of the second half of the alphabet, excepting n, which was used for mathematical equations and O, which Einthoven used to mark the beginning of each recording he made. The U wave was not discovered until 1906.

P Wave

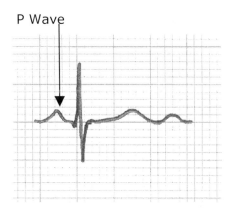

The P wave is the first deflection of the normal cardiac electrical cycle. It represents atrial depolarization.

Characteristics

Location: First deflection of the cardiac cycle, precedes the QRS complex

Amplitude: Less than 2-3 mm

Duration: 0.08-0.11 sec

Contour: Rounded and upright in leads I, II, aVF, and V_1 –V_6; can be positive, negative or biphasic in III, V_1-V_3, and aVL; should be negative in aVR.

Importance: Indicates the firing of the SA node, the normal pacemaker for the heart. The P waves should all look alike.

Abnormalities: Flat P waves indicate left atrial hypertrophy, while peaked P waves occur with right atrial hypertrophy. Enlargement of the P wave may be indicative of conditions such as mitral stenosis or

COPD. Inverted P waves can indicate a retrograde firing from a pacemaker site other than the SA node.

P-R Interval

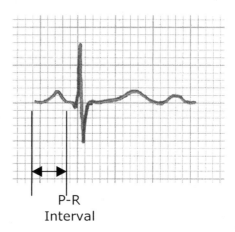

P-R Interval

The P-R Interval is the portion of the tracing from the beginning of the P wave to the beginning of the QRS complex. It represents atrial depolarization plus the time it takes for an impulse to travel from the SA node, through the atria, the AV node, bundle of His and to the Purkinje fibers. Depolarization of the AV node, bundle of His, bundle branches and the Purkinje fibers are to small in amplitude to be detected by surface electrodes.

> **Characteristics**
>> **Location:** Starts at the beginning of the P wave and extends to the beginning of the QRS complex
>> **Amplitude:** N/A
>> **Duration:** 0.12 – 0.20 sec
>> **Contour:** P wave should be well rounded and the PR segment should flat (isolectric).

Importance: Signifies the normal progression of the electrical impulse through the cardiac fibers. Used to determine AV blocks.

Abnormalities: Short P-R intervals are associated with junctional rhythms and in pre-excitation syndromes or re-entry type tachycardias. Longer P-R intervals are noted in the presence of arteriosclerosis, inflammation, hypoxia, scarring, drug toxicities, and first degree AV block. Elevated PR intervals are noted with atrial infections and pericarditis.

QRS Complex

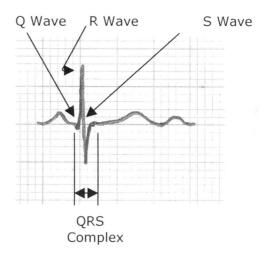

QRS Complex

The QRS complex is actually made up of three separate waves occurring closely together as the electrical impulse travels through the ventricles. Both ventricles are simultaneously activated, but, since the left ventricle is somewhat thicker, it requires a slightly longer time to conduct the impulse. The QRS complex represents ventricular depolarization. The first downward deflection of the complex is labeled the Q wave; the first upward deflection is the R wave, and the first upward deflection **following** the R wave is the S wave. All positive waves of the QRS complex are labeled R waves; the first R, the next R', etc. Negative waves occurring before the R wave are labeled Q, and those afterward S. Subsequent deflections are labeled S_1, S_2, etc. Some experts will label waves larger than 5mm with upper case letters, and waves smaller than 4mm with lower case letters. In some instances, not all waves are discernable, but the complex is referred to as the QRS complex. It is measured from the beginning of the Q wave to the end of the S wave.

Characteristics

    Location: Immediately follows P-R interval

    Amplitude: Varies, but should gradually become taller, then gradually shorten across the V leads, with V_4 or V_5 being the tallest. The waves should be taller than 6mm, but should not be taller than 25-30mm in the chest leads

    Duration: 0.04 – 0.12 seconds. The widest QRS measurement on the 12 lead EKG is considered the correct one.

    Contour: May look different in each lead. Positively deflected in Leads I, II, III, aVL, aVF, V_{4-6}, Negatively deflected in Leads aVR, V_1, V_2, and may be biphasic in Leads V_3 and V_4. The QRS complex is best viewed in leads I and V_1.

    Importance: Signifies passage of the electrical impulse through the Purkinje system.

Abnormalities: Smaller than normal complexes may be seen in patients with cardiac failure, diffuse coronary artery disease, pericardial effusions, myxedema, emphysema, generalized edema, and obesity. Wider complexes (greater than 0.12 sec) are sometimes seen when the impulse is slowed through one of the ventricles, such as bundle branch blocks and premature ventricular systoles. "Early" R waves – those as tall in V_1 and V_2 as the next several leads - can signify a posterior, or lateral wall infarction, right ventricular hypertrophy, or Wolfe-Parkinson-White Syndrome.

Q Wave

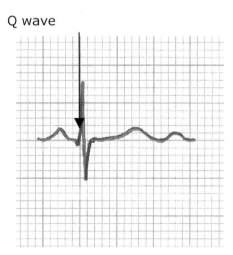
Q wave

The Q wave is the negative wave preceding the R wave. Not all leads record a Q wave. Normal Q waves represent septal depolarization, but they must be distinguished from pathologic Q waves, which signify an infarction. A pathological Q wave is 0.04 sec (1 box wide) and higher than 1/3 the amplitude of the QRS complex as seen in lead III.

Characteristics

Location: The first negative deflection preceding the R wave. Normal Q waves are present only in Leads I, aVL, V_5 and V_6.

Amplitude: Not deeper than 1/3 the height of the QRS complex

Duration: Should be less than 0.04 seconds

Importance: Large Q waves represent myocardial damage

J Point

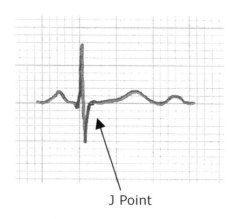

J Point

The J point represents the end of the QRS complex, and the beginning of the ST segment. The JT interval (measured from the J point to the beginning of the T wave) reflects repolarization alone. It is sometimes used to measure the refractory period of patients on sodium channel blockers. Those drugs slow depolarization and slightly prolong the QRS complex.

ST Segment

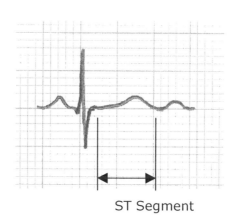

ST Segment

The ST segment represents the end of ventricular depolarization and marks the beginning of ventricular repolarization; a time when the ventricles are in their absolute refractory period and will not respond to stimuli. It is usually isolectric, but may deviate above or below the baseline.

Characteristics

Location: Extends from the end of the QRS complex (the J point) to the beginning of the S wave.

Amplitude: Usually isolectric, but may be seen above or below baseline.

Duration: The duration of the ST segment varies greatly, but is usually not measured as a part of the interpretation of the rhythm.

Contour: Usually varies less than 1mm from the isolectric line in either direction.

Importance: Represents the beginning to the ventricular repolarization process.

Abnormalities: Elevation of 2mm or more is seen with myocardial injury or infarction. Depression of 2mm or greater is seen with episodes of myocardial ischemia. Conditions such as pulmonary emboli, pericarditis, left ventricular hypertrophy, myocarditis, and medications such as digoxin and Amiodarone may also have an effect on the ST segment. ST segment changes are usually transient.

T Wave

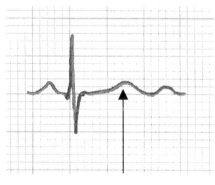

T Wave

The T wave represents ventricular repolarization. It is the first wave following the QRS complex and ST segment.

Characteristics

Location: Wave immediately following ST segment

Amplitude: 5mm or less in the limb leads and 10mm or less in the chest leads

Duration: Not measured individually, but included in the measurement of the QT interval.

Contour: Normally smoothly rounded upright in Leads I, II, V_3 – V_6; inverted in aVR; and may be upright or inverted in Leads III, V_1, V_2, aVL, and aVF, depending upon the hearts electrical position. It should have the same polarity as the QRS complex. Food intake and certain drugs can affect the T wave.

Importance: Represents the vulnerable point of repolarization; a point where the hearts rhythm can be affected by undesired stimuli, usually coinciding with the apex of the T wave.

Abnormalities: T wave inversion is indicative of myocardial ischemia; peaked T waves are seen with hyperkalemia, and notched T waves can indicate pericarditis. T waves are not as reliable as ST elevation or depression in the diagnosis of ischemia. Other factors that may influence the T wave include: age; especially juveniles, CVA; particularly ones with intra cranial bleeding, post tachycardia or pacemaker rhythms, intermittent left bundle branch blocks, cardiomyopathy, Wolfe-Parkinson-White Syndrome, and respiratory alkalosis

QT Interval

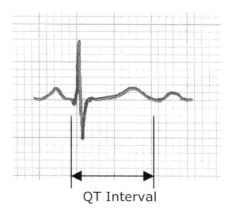

QT Interval

The QT interval represents the time required for ventricular depolarization and repolarization. During this time, the ventricles have responded the electrical stimuli passed through from the AV node, and have returned to the "ready" state, awaiting the next impulse.

Characteristics

Location: The QT interval is measured from the beginning of the QRS complex to the end of the T wave. It is best viewed in leads V_2 or V_3.

Amplitude: Not measured

Duration: Varies according to heart rate, shortening with faster heart rates and increasing with slower rates but generally 0.36 – 0.44 sec if the heart rate is 60. For heart rates greater than 60 the QTc (QT corrected) is 0.44 sec. To calculate the QTc: divide the QT interval (in seconds) by the square root of the R-R interval (in seconds).

$$QTc = \frac{QT\ interval}{\sqrt{R\text{-}R\ interval}}$$

Contour: Not measured

Importance: Represents ventricular refractory time; the time the ventricles are susceptible to outside stimuli.

Abnormalities: Medications such as digitalis and potassium, or rhythms such as sinus tachycardia may shorten the QT interval, while certain anti-arrhythmics, bradycardias, and hereditary conditions may prolong it.

U Wave

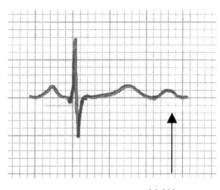

U Wave

The U wave is a small deflection sometimes noticed after or immediately superimposed on the T wave. The exact reason for the U wave is unknown, but it is believed to represent repolarization of the Purkinje fibers. It may also be seen when serum potassium levels are low, or during bradycardia.

Characteristics

Location: Immediately following or superimposed onto the T wave

Amplitude: Not measured

Duration: Not measured

Contour: Generally deflected the same direction as the T wave.

Importance: Believed to represent the repolarization of the Purkinje fibers

Abnormalities: Negative deflection may be seen in patients with left ventricular hypertrophy, hypertension and coronary artery disease. An upwardly deflected U wave that peaks during exercise stress may indicate significant obstruction in the left anterior descending coronary artery.

Calculating the Rate

Knowing that time is constant, one can easily calculate the rate from an EKG tracing. This can be done using one of several methods or with a marked device.

A. Division - If the heart rate is regular, count the number of large boxes between two consecutive QRS complexes and divide 300 by that number. Example: the complexes are three large boxes apart. 300 ÷ 3 = 100. The heart rate is approximately 100. For a more precise rate, divide 1500 by the number of small boxes between two consecutive complexes.

B. If the heart rate is irregular- Obtain a six second tracing, count the number of complexes and multiply that number by 10. (Six seconds times ten equals one minute)

C. Sequence Method- Find a complex that occurs on a dark line. Count the next dark lines as follows: 300, 150, 100, 75, 60, 50, 42, 37... ending with the number of the dark line closes to the next complex. This is an approximate rate.

D. Rate calculator cards- Place the card over the rhythm strip, align the indicator mark with a QRS complex, and read the rate as per the instructions on the card.

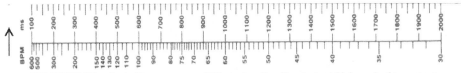

HEART RATE (25mm/sec) Place arrow on a QRS complex. Read heart rate at third complex from arrow.

HEART RATE AND TIME INTERVAL CALCULATION TABLE

Number of Small Squares	Rate	Time (sec.)	Number of Small Squares	Rate	Time (sec.)
2	750	0.08	27	55	1.08
4	375	0.16	28	54	1.12
5	300	0.20	29	52	1.16
6	250	0.24	30	50	1.20
7	214	0.28	31	48	1.24
8	188	0.32	32	47	1.28
9	168	0.36	33	45	1.32
10	150	0.40	34	44	1.36
11	136	0.44	35	43	1.40
12	125	0.48	36	42	1.44
13	115	0.52	37	41	1.48
14	107	0.56	38	40	1.52
15	100	0.60	39	39	1.56
16	94	0.64	40	38	1.60
17	88	0.68	42	36	1.68
18	83	0.72	44	35	1.76
19	79	0.76	46	33	1.84
20	75	0.80	48	31	1.92
21	72	0.84	50	30	2
22	68	0.88	52	29	2.08
23	65	0.92	54	28	2.16
24	63	0.96	56	27	2.24
25	60	1	58	26	2.32
26	58	1.04	60	25	2.40

Chapter Four

From the Top

Atrial Rhythms

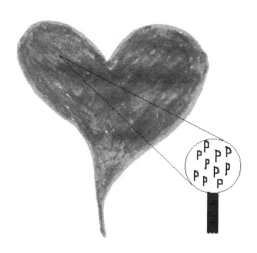

SINUS RHYTHM

ATRIAL

    RATE   60 – 100
                         P-R-Interval   0.12-0.20 sec.

    RHYTHM Regular
                         P-P interval may vary slightly, but not more than 0.16 seconds

    CONTOUR Normal (rounded, symmetrical)
                         P waves occur upright in leads **I, II, II**

VENTRICULAR

    RATE   60–100
                         Q-T Interval 0.28-0.48 sec.

    RHYTHM Regular
                         R-R interval may vary slightly, but not more than 0.16 seconds

    CONTOUR Normal
                         QRS complex is narrow, no wider than 0.12 seconds

CHARACTERISTICS

- ♥ Normal Sinus Rhythm **(NSR)** is the most common adult rhythm.
- ♥ The pacemaker site is the SA node.

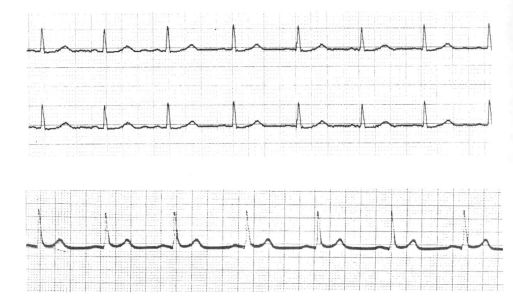

SINUS BRADYCARDIA

ATRIAL

- **RATE** — Less than 60
  PRI 0.12-0.20 sec

- **RHYTHM** — Regular
  P-P interval may vary slightly, but not more than 0.16 seconds

- **CONTOUR** — Normal
  P waves occur upright in leads **I, II, II**

VENTRICULAR

- **RATE** — Less than 60
  QTI 0.28-0.48 sec

- **RHYTHM** — Regular
  R-R interval may vary slightly, but not more than 0.16 seconds

- **CONTOUR** — Normal
  QRS complex is narrow, no wider than 0.12 seconds

CHARACTERISTICS

- ♥ Sinus Bradycardia can be normal in some individuals, such as well-trained athletes. Non-cardiac causes include: increased ocular pressure, increased intracranial pressure, obstructive jaundice (bile salts will affect the SA node), hypothermia and hyperkalemia.

CAUSES

- ♥ Excessive vagal tone
- ♥ Decreased sympathetic tone
- ♥ Myocardial infarction
- ♥ Medication overdoses such as digitalis, and morphine.

- ♥ This rhythm is usually benign, but it may compromise myocardial function in patients with inferior or posterior infarctions.

TREATMENT

- ♥ None required for the asymptomatic patient.
- ♥ Atropine and pacing are indicated if symptoms present.

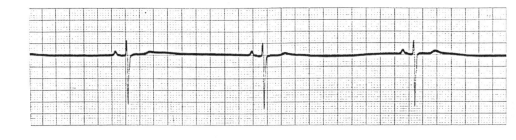

SINUS TACHYCARDIA

ATRIAL

- **RATE** 100-180

- **RHYTHM** Regular
  P-P interval may vary slightly, but not more than 0.16 seconds

- **CONTOUR** Normal
  P waves occur upright in leads **I, II, II**

VENTRICULAR

- **RATE** 100-180

- **RHYTHM** Regular
  R-R interval may vary slightly, but not more than 0.16 seconds

- **CONTOUR** Normal
  QRS complex is narrow, no wider than 0.12 seconds

CHARACTERISTICS

Sinus tachycardia will usually have a gradual onset and termination. Vagal maneuvers will usually slow and restore a normal rhythm.

CAUSES

- ♥ Increased sympathetic stimulation caused by factors such as: pain, fever, hypotension, anemia, anxiety, hypovolemia, pulmonary embolus, myocardial ischemia, shock, certain infections, stimulants such as caffeine, and tobacco.
- ♥ The tachycardia may be related to angina, and possibly tend to cause an increase in the size of an infarction.

TREATMENT

- ♥ Find and treat underlying cause

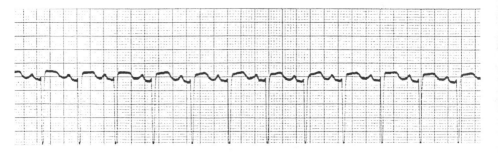

SUPRAVENTRICULAR TACHYCARDIA

PSVT

ATRIAL

- **RATE** 150-250

- **RHYTHM** Regular
  Pacemaker site is an ectopic focus in the atria

- **CONTOUR** Retrograde, flattened, notched, or biphasic. Sometimes lost in the QRS complex.
  The P wave may be abnormally shaped, or not visible at all due to the fact it may be buried in the QRS complex.

VENTRICULAR

- **RATE** 150-250

- **RHYTHM** Regular
  R-R interval may vary slightly, but not more than 0.16 seconds
  R-R interval may shorten during the first few beats, and lengthen during the last few beats of the arrhythmia

- **CONTOUR** Normal
  QRS complex is narrow, no wider than 0.12 seconds

CHARACTERISTICS

- ♥ **Rapid regular tachycardia with sudden onset and termination**
- ♥ It may sometimes be seen starting after a premature atrial event, which contains a prolonged PR interval.
- ♥ Abrupt termination is sometimes followed by a brief period of asystole
- ♥ Patients usually report a sudden onset of fluttering or pounding in the chest

accompanied with feelings of weakness and shortness of breath. Myocardial oxygen needs increase, cardiac output decreases, and insufficient filling of the heart results from the rapidness of the tachycardia.
♥ Stable patients may rapidly deteriorate if the arrhythmia is not terminated.

CAUSES

♥ PSVT is most commonly caused by an A-V nodal reentry, or reentry over an accessory pathway

TREATMENT

♥ **Stimulation of the Vagus nerve** through measures such as: carotid sinus massage, gagging, rectal stimulation, massaging the eyeball.
♥ **Valsalva maneuver**, which will increase intrathoracic pressure, decrease venous return, increase the blood pressure, and slow the heart.
♥ **Medications,** such as Adenosine, Calcium channel blockers, Beta-blockers, Digoxin.
♥ **Electrical Cardioversion**

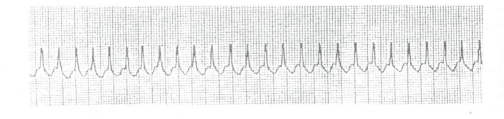

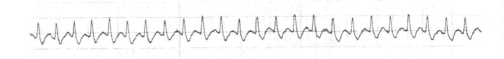

Supraventricular -meaning above the ventricles, can include any of the rapid complex tachycardias, including the old name PAT, which is no longer used unless P waves are clearly seen; Atrial fibrillation, Atrial flutter, Junctional tachycardia, Accelerated junctional rhythm, and Multifocal atrial tachycardia. The rhythm is named PSVT if the onset and termination are seen.

SINUS ARRHYTHMIA

ATRIAL

    RATE   50-100
                       PRI < 0.20 sec

    RHYTHM   Irregular, characterized by a phasic variation in cycle length of greater than 0.16 seconds.

    CONTOUR   Normal

VENTRICULAR

    RATE   50-100
                       QTI 0.36-0.44 sec

    RHYTHM   Irregular

    CONTOUR   Normal
                       QRS complex is narrow, no wider than 0.12 seconds

CHARACTERISTICS

- Two basic forms are noted; respiratory and non-respiratory. In the respiratory form, the P-P interval varies with respirations, increasing with inspiration and decreasing with expiration due to rhythmic fluctuations in vagal tone. In the non-respiratory form, the same phasic pattern, but it does not correlate with the respiratory pattern.

CAUSES

- Exact causes are unknown, but the arrhythmia is more commonly seen in the young and in elderly patients.

TREATMENT

♥ No treatment is required. Exercise will usually increase the heart rate significantly.

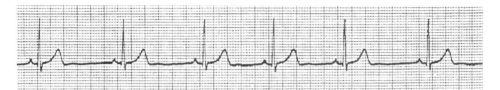

SINUS ARREST

ATRIAL

RATE	60-100 **PRI** <0.20 sec	
RHYTHM	May be regular or irregular	
CONTOUR	Normal except where absent	

VENTRICULAR

RATE	60-100 **QTI** 0.36-0.44 sec	
RHYTHM	Usually regular except where complex is dropped	
CONTOUR	Contour and QT interval are normal	

CHARACTERISTICS
- ♥ P-P interval usually will not be twice the normal interval.
- ♥ The timing mechanism is reset and the entire complex is dropped.
- ♥ There is no QRS complex since no P wave was fired
- ♥ Atrial escape complexes may occur during periods of sinus arrest.
  - ♥ Characterized by a P wave that occurs later than would be expected.
  - ♥ Occur only when the normal pacemaker does not function

CAUSES
- ♥ Failure of the SA node to discharge
- ♥ Involvement of the SA node or sinus node artery by an MI,
- ♥ Drug toxicity (digoxin, salycilates, quinidine, beta blockers, some calcium channel blockers),

- ♥ Excessive vagal tone
- ♥ Certain forms of fibrosis

TREATMENT

- ♥ No treatment is required for the asymptomatic patient.
- ♥ Atropine and pacing are indicated for the symptomatic patient.

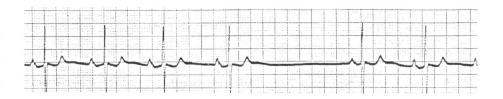

SINUS BLOCK/ SINO-ATRIAL BLOCK

ATRIAL

    RATE   60-100
                    PRI <0.20 sec

    RHYTHM   Regular

    CONTOUR   Normal

VENTRICULAR

    RATE   60-100
                    QTI 0.36-0.44

    RHYTHM   Regular

    CONTOUR   Normal

CHARACTERISTICS
- An impulse is formed in the SA node, but is blocked from depolarizing the atria
- The normally expected P wave is absent, and therefore no QRS T follows, basically, an entire cycle is "just missing."
- The P-P internal is usually a multiple of the basic P-P interval.
- It can be manifested as occasional dropped beats to no P waves at all (short periods of asystole).

CAUSES
- Excessive vagal stimulation
- Acute infections
- Fibrosis involving the atrium
- MI
- Myocardial ischemia
- Sinus node ischemia or infarction
- Degenerative changes associated with aging
- Drugs such as atropine, salycilates, procainamide, and digoxin

There are four known explanations for the absence of P waves:

1. Failure of the SA node to form the impulse (generator failure)
2. Failure of the impulse to discharge from the node (exit block)
3. Atrial paralysis, as seen with potassium intoxication
4. Sinus impulses too weak to activate the atria

TREATMENT
- Sinus block is usually transient and is of no clinical significance.
- Symptomatic bradycardia may be treated with Atropine and pacing.

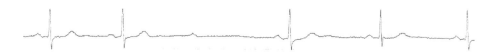

SICK SINUS SYNDROME

Sick Sinus Syndrome is not a particular rhythm, but a pattern which manifests itself as:
- Episodes of marked sinus bradycardia or sinus arrest resistant to atropine
- Longer pauses up to 12 seconds following events such as:
  - PAC
  - Spontaneous conversion from atrial fibrillation or atrial flutter
  - Rapid atrial overdrive pacing
  - DC cardioversion

Symptoms may include palpitations, syncope, congestive heart failure and angina.

Sick sinus syndrome can co-exist with atrial fibrillation and atrial flutter in elderly patients.

CAUSES
- The same as those leading to sinus bradycardia and sinus arrest:
- Vagal events
- Acute infections
- Fibrosis involving the atrium
- Drugs
- Degenerative changes associated with aging

TREATMENT
- Permanent pacemaker implantation followed by medications to control any tachycardic rhythms.

73

PREMATURE ATRIAL CONTRACTIONS
PAC

Not a rhythm but an event

ATRIAL

    RATE

        PRI 0.12-0.20 in normal beats, but may vary in ectopics

    RHYTHM   Premature

    CONTOUR Abnormal

VENTRICULAR

    RATE

        QTI 0.36-0.44

    RHYTHM   Irregular

    CONTOUR Normal

CHARACTERISTICS

- ♥ Premature P wave followed by a normal QRS complex
- ♥ The irregular P wave may sometimes be difficult to distinguish when it is superimposed on the preceding T wave.
- ♥ The cycle following the PAC is usually slightly longer than the dominant sinus cycle, but less than a full compensatory pause.
- ♥ The AV junction may still be refractory from the preceding beat and may prevent conduction of the beat resulting in a blocked PAC, which is common.
- ♥ The PAC will be conducted normally, conducted aberrantly, or not conducted at all. Dr. Marriott, a pioneer in arrhythmia recognition, observed, "The commonest causes of pauses are non-conducted PACs."

- ♥ Conduction will be normal if the PAC arrives at the AV junction after it is repolarized. It will be aberrant if the impulse reaches the His-Purkinje system while one or both are in its refractory period, with QRS complexes being wider and resembling a bundle branch block pattern.
- ♥ PACs in leads V1 and V6 usually appear triphasic and predominately positively deflected, and may look similar to PVCs, therefore diagnosis should focus on finding a preceding P wave.
- ♥ PACs will usually reset the P-P cycle.

Variations include:

- ♥ Atrial couplets – two PACs in a row
- ♥ Multifocal atrial couplets – two PACs in a row, but having P waves of different morphologies

Both are unusual and benign, but in the presence of pulmonary disease, increase the susceptibility to MAT, A fib, and A flutter.

CAUSES

- ♥ PACs are normal findings in adults,
- ♥ Atrial irritability
- ♥ Stress
- ♥ Fatigue
- ♥ Stimulants such as nicotine and caffeine
- ♥ Alcohol
- ♥ Hyperthyroidism
- ♥ Post MI
- ♥ CHF
- ♥ Acute respiratory failure
- ♥ COPD
- ♥ Electrolyte imbalances
- ♥ Hypoxia
- ♥ Digitalis toxicity
- ♥ PACs may be warning signs of more serious arrhythmias

TREATMENT
- Eliminate causes
- Administer drugs that prolong atrial refractoriness, such as Procainamide, and Verapamil.

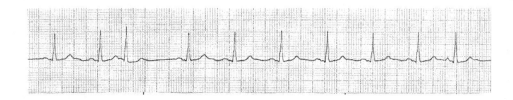

PAC's can also be blocked. The impulse is generated in the SA node, but is blocked from being transmitted through the AV junction and through the ventricles. An early P wave can usually be seen.

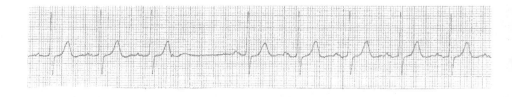

WANDERING ATRIAL PACEMAKER
WAP

ATRIAL

- **RATE**   50-150
  PRI varies according to pacemaker location

- **RHYTHM**   Irregular

- **CONTOUR**   Irregular

VENTRICULAR

- **RATE**   50-150
  QTI 0.36-0.44

- **RHYTHM**   Irregular

- **CONTOUR**   Normal

CHARACTERISTICS
- ♥ A variation of Sinus Arrhythmia
- ♥ The dominant pacemaker site is transferred to various sites within the atrial or AV junctional tissue.
- ♥ Only one pacemaker site is operative at a time, and **changes occur gradually** over the course of several beats
- ♥ This arrhythmia is more commonly seen with narrow complex rhythms around 60 beats per minute

CAUSES
- ♥ This may be a normal phenomenon in young, elderly and highly athletic individuals,
- ♥ May be a manifestation of fluctuating vagal tone.

TREATMENT

♥ No treatment is required, as this is a benign rhythm.

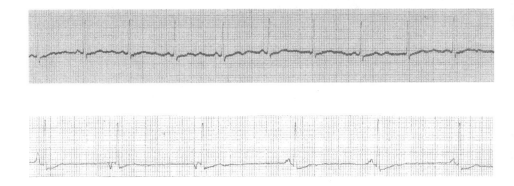

ATRIAL TACHYCARDIA

ATRIAL

RATE		150-250
		PRI May increase until a 2:1 conduction pattern occurs
RHYTHM		Regular
CONTOUR		Abnormal

VENTRICULAR

RATE		75-200 varies with degree of conduction
		QTI 0.36-0.44
RHYTHM		Generally regular
CONTOUR		Normal

CHARACTERISTICS

- ♥ In about 50% of all cases the atrial rate is irregular, whereas in PSVT (Paroxysmal Supra Ventricular Tachycardia) it is extremely regular.
- ♥ This rhythm is commonly misdiagnosed as atrial flutter. Atrial tachycardia has **distinguishable P waves**. Atrial flutter has **sawtooth** flutter waves at a faster rate.

CAUSES

- ♥ Coronary artery disease
- ♥ Cor Pulmonale
- ♥ Digoxin excess
- ♥ Autonomic atrial foci
- ♥ Re-entry circuit within the atrium

TREATMENT

- ♥ For patients with a slow ventricular rate with a block: atropine
- ♥ Fast rate: Carotid Sinus Massage, Adenosine, DC Cardioversion.

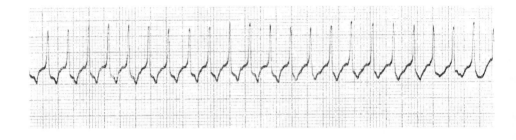

MULTIFOCAL ATRIAL TACHYCARDIA
MAT

ATRIAL

    RATE   100-250
                    PRI Varies

    RHYTHM   Irregular

    CONTOUR   Irregular

VENTRICULAR

    RATE   100-250
                    QTI 0.36-0.44

    RHYTHM   Irregular

    CONTOUR   Normal

CHARACTERISTICS

- ♥ MAT is similar to atrial tachycardia, but with a marked variation in P wave morphology, and P-P interval. Several different pacemaker sites within the atria are each firing at near normal rates, but the ventricular rate is usually tachycardic as a response to the multiple atrial impulses being conducted. Rapid ventricular rates may lead to hypotension, angina or congestive heart failure.

CAUSES

- ♥ Two or more asynchronous atrial pacemakers are responsible for MAT.
- ♥ It usually occurs in persons over the age of 50, and is exacerbated by respiratory failure, hypertension, hypokalemia, hypomagnesaemia, and has been associated with elderly patients,

- critically ill patients and those with diabetes.
- ♥ Found more frequently in males than females.
- ♥ Rarely produced by digitalis

TREATMENT

- ♥ Exercise or sinus tachycardia can usually break this rhythm. An increase in the rate of discharge of the sinus node will usually over pace the ectopic pacemakers. Improving lung function can be helpful.
- ♥ Verapamil will sometimes reduce the heart rate and suppress the firing of abnormal pacemaker cells.

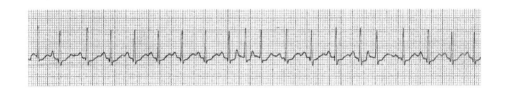

ATRIAL FIBRILLATION
Af

ATRIAL

    RATE   400-600
                      PRI None

    RHYTHM   Irregular

    CONTOUR   No identifiable P waves are present. Instead fibrillitory waves are present, which vary in amplitude. They can best be seen in leads I, II, and aVF.

VENTRICULAR

    RATE   60-160
                      QTI Normal, but difficult to measure due to overlying fibrillitory waves

    RHYTHM   Irregularly irregular

    CONTOUR   Normal

CHARACTERISTICS

- ♥ Atrial fibrillation represents a total disorganization of atrial activity without an effective atrial contraction.
- ♥ Ventricular response is totally irregular, but is easier to slow than atrial flutter due to the lack of organization of the impulses.
- ♥ Chances of forming an atrial thrombus are greatly increased after the first 48 hours of this rhythm due to the fact that the atrial filling is only 20-30% of normal.
- ♥ The term "controlled" is used when the ventricular rate remains under 100. V1 is the best lead for identifying atrial activity.
- ♥ Atrial fibrillation is the most common supraventricular rhythm, found in 4 out of

100 patients 55-64 years old, and 9 out of 100 patients over 65.
- ♥ It is found more frequently in males than females.
- ♥ In the presence of an accessory pathway, atrial fibrillation can have rapid, irregular, wide QRS complexes, which can resemble ventricular tachycardia.
- ♥ Atrial fibrillation should be suspected in younger hemodynamically stable patients. Look for the irregularly irregular R-R interval.

Obtain a 12 lead EKG for confirmation if an accessory pathway rhythm is suspected—Digitalis given in the presence of an accessory pathway can actually accelerate conduction through that pathway.

CAUSES
- ♥ Digoxin toxicity
- ♥ Mitral stenosis
- ♥ Cardiomyopathy
- ♥ Hypertensive heart disease
- ♥ Coronary artery disease
- ♥ Pericarditis
- ♥ COPD
- ♥ CHF
- ♥ May be precipitated by a period of excessive alcohol consumption.
- ♥ The rhythm can be chronic or paroxysmal

TREATMENT
- ♥ Digoxin,
- ♥ DC cardioversion
- ♥ Catheter ablation with pacemaker insertion
- ♥ Carotid sinus massage will only slow the ventricular response, but the rhythm will remain irregular.
- ♥ Lidocaine and Procainamide given in the presence of atrial fibrillation can actually increase the rate due to a change in the conduction ratio.

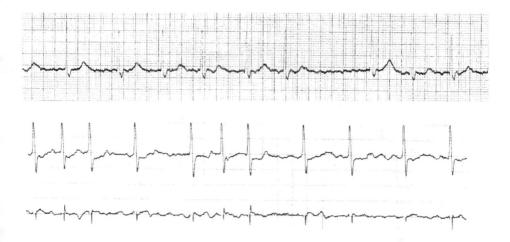

ATRIAL FLUTTER
AF

ATRIAL

- **RATE**   250-350
  PRI None

- **RHYTHM**   Regular

- **CONTOUR**   Saw-toothed. Called F (flutter) waves. Best seen in leads II, III, aVF, and V1

VENTRICULAR

- **RATE**   75-175 (1/2 or less of the atrial rate)

- **RHYTHM**   Generally regular

- **CONTOUR**   Normal
  QT Difficult to identify

CHARACTERISTICS

- ♥ Identically regular saw tooth flutter waves replace P waves.
- ♥ Best seen in leads II, III, and aVF.
- ♥ Usually there is a fixed conduction ratio with 2:1 being the most common. 4:1 is the next most common, while odd numbered ratios 3:1, 5:1, etc. are rare.
- ♥ A second type of Atrial Flutter, with ventricular rates greater than 350 beats per minute, is known. It is difficult to treat and often converts to ventricular fibrillation.

CAUSES

- ♥ Inferior wall MI
- ♥ Mitral or tricuspid valve disease
- ♥ Cor pulmonale
- ♥ Sick Sinus Syndrome
- ♥ Hypertension
- ♥ Cardiomegaly

- ♥ COPD
- ♥ Hyperthyroidism
- ♥ Hypoxia
- ♥ Pericarditis
- ♥ Atrial flutter is a reentry circuit type rhythm, beginning with a premature beat, which may be acute or chronic.
- ♥ Most common in persons over 40 years of age with ischemic heart disease.

TREATMENT

- ♥ Cardioversion
- ♥ Atrial overdrive pacing
- ♥ Drugs such as Lidocaine, Procainamide, and Quinidine can actually increase the ventricular rate due to a change in the conduction ratio.

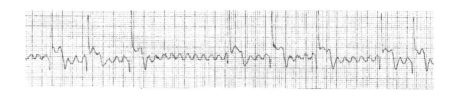

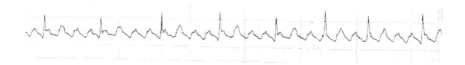

Chapter 5

In the Middle

Junctional Rhythms

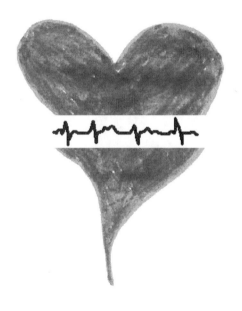

JUNCTIONAL RHYTHM

ATRIAL

- **RATE** <40
  PRI Less than 0.12 sec. if measurable.

- **RHYTHM** Regular

- **CONTOUR** Regular. May precede, be buried within, or follow the QRS complex. P waves are inverted in II, III, and aVF.

VENTRICULAR

- **RATE** 40-60
  QTI 0.36-0.44

- **RHYTHM** Regular

- **CONTOUR** May be abnormal, but less than 0.12 sec. wide.

CHARACTERISTICS

- ♥ Junctional rhythm is an escape rhythm originating in the Bundle of His.
- ♥ It acts as a safety mechanism to control the cardiac rhythm and prevent the occurrence of ventricular asystole.
- ♥ It may precipitate the occurrence of sustained ventricular tachycardia.
- ♥ The first beat of a junctional escape rhythm occurs later in the cycle than the normal beat would be expected.

CAUSES

- ♥ Infection
- ♥ Inflammation
- ♥ Myocardial ischemia
- ♥ Sick sinus syndrome
- ♥ Tobacco

- ♥ Caffeine
- ♥ Medications such as digitalis
- ♥ It may be a normal response due to vagal effect on the higher pacemaker, or may occur during a pathologic slow sinus discharge.

TREATMENT

- ♥ Increase the discharge rate of the higher pacemaker.
- ♥ Atropine is the drug of choice for symptomatic bradycardia.
- ♥ Pacing is rarely needed.

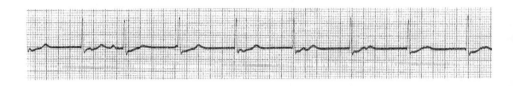

PREMATURE JUNCTIONAL CONTRACTIONS
PJC

ATRIAL

    RATE   N/A
                      PRI <0.12 sec.

    RHYTHM   Irregular

    CONTOUR   P waves are of the opposite from normal deflection in leads I, II, III, aVf, and V6. P waves may be abnormal, and be shortly preceding, buried within, or less commonly closely following the QRS complex.

VENTRICULAR

    RATE
                      QTI 0.36-0.44

    RHYTHM   Irregular

    CONTOUR   May be abnormal, but <0.122 sec.

CHARACTERISTICS

- A premature systole occurs from the AV junction and spreads retrograde to the atrium producing a premature, abnormal P wave. This is commonly followed by a compensatory pause unless the atria and AV junction fire at the same time.
- PJCs are much less common than PACs or PVCs.

CAUSES

- Digitalis toxicity is the most common cause.
- MI
- Ischemia
- Caffeine
- Amphetamines
- Irritable focus in the AV junction

- ♥ Enhanced automaticity in junctional tissue within the Bundle of His.
- ♥ The exact origin of the beat is difficult to distinguish from the surface EKG.
- ♥ Frequent PJCs can produce junctional tachycardia, a more dangerous arrhythmia.

TREATMENT

- ♥ This is usually a benign occurrence and no treatment is required.
- ♥ Atropine and pacing may be used in for symptomatic bradycardias.
- ♥ PJCs are unusual in healthy individuals.
- ♥ Suspect that the arrhythmia may be atrial in nature if the person has no underlying cardiac disorder.

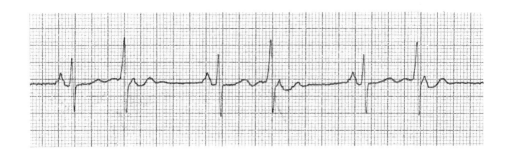

ACCELERATED JUNCTIONAL RHYTHM & JUNCTIONAL TACHYCARDIA

ATRIAL

    RATE   **AJR** 60-100   **JT** >100-250
                PRI <0.12 sec. if measurable

    RHYTHM   Regular

    CONTOUR   P waves inverted or absent

VENTRICULAR

    RATE   **AJR** 60-100   **JT** >100-250
                QT Normal

    RHYTHM   Regular

    CONTOUR   Normal

Tachycardia, by definition, is generally thought of as rates greater than 100 beats per minute. The normal rate for junctional rhythms is 40 to 60 beats per minute. Since the rate of this rhythm is above what is considered normal, the rhythm is labeled tachycardia.

CHARACTERISTICS
- Gradual onset and termination
- Often a transient rhythm
- Junctional tachycardia is an early sign of digitalis toxicity in a patient with atrial fibrillation.
- This rhythm may decrease cardiac output by decreasing ventricular filling.

CAUSES
- An ectopic foci in the Bundle of His
- Digitalis toxicity
- Hypoxia
- Acute Rheumatic fever
- Postoperative valve symptoms
- Myocarditis
- Cardiomyopathy

- ♥ Myocardial infarctions

TREATMENT

- ♥ It is important to distinguish these rhythms from ventricular tachycardia, as the treatments differ.
- ♥ Vagal maneuvers
- ♥ Adenosine
- ♥ Cardioversion
- ♥ Rapid atrial overdrive pacing may be employed to slow this rhythm.
- ♥ Radio frequency ablation is used to disable the ectopic foci.

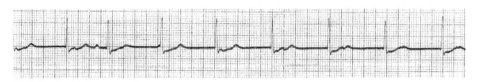

AV Nodal Re-entrant Tachycardia (AVNRT) is a reentry tachycardia occurring within or near the AV node. The normal heart has two separate pathways leading to a common AV node. Impulses normally traverse both pathways simultaneously. Ischemia can slow conduction through one of the pathways, which increases the chance of the impulse reaching the AV node at different times. When this occurs, the impulse will normally be conducted down the slower pathway to the ventricles, and may then follow the faster conducting pathway back to the atria, allowing for a tachycardic rhythm. This occurs in approximately 20% of all narrow complex tachycardias.

Chapter Six

From the Bottom

Ventricular Rhythms

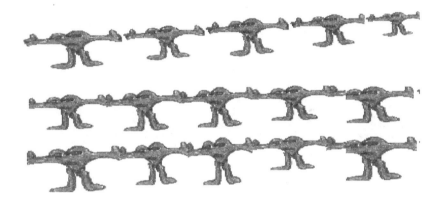

PREMATURE VENTRICULAR COMPLEXES
PVC

PVCs are an event rather than a rhythm. They may or may not affect atrial activity.

ATRIAL

    RATE

    RHYTHM

    CONTOUR

VENTRICULAR

    RATE

    RHYTHM

    CONTOUR   A wide, bizarre QRS complex with the T wave usually occurring opposite the normal deflection

CHARACTERISTICS

- ♥ PVCs are the most common dysrhythmia, seen in 50-63% of healthy individuals, and 72-93% of post MI patients.
- ♥ Characterized by a wide, bizarre QRS complex occurring early in the cycle
- ♥ The PVC is generally not preceded by a P wave, but one may be seen as a result of the SA node firing in it's normal cycle.
- ♥ Retrograde conduction does occur, but retrograde P waves are rarely seen.
- ♥ PVCs are commonly followed by a compensatory pause, however, if a retrograde impulse discharges the sinus node prematurely and resets the timing mechanism, an incomplete compensatory pause may result.

A compensatory pause occurs when the premature systole does not reset the timing mechanism allowing the impulse to be fired from the SA node at its normal time. The impulse does not reach the ventricle since the tissue has not yet repolarized from the premature ventricular systole. The R-R interval produced by the two complexes equals twice that of the normally conducted R-R interval.

An interpolated PVC is one that occurs without causing a compensatory pause. The sinus complex after the PVC may be conducted with a prolonged PR interval.

A ventricular fusion beat is produced by simultaneous firing of the ventricular systole and a normal sinus beat. This indicates the ventricle has been depolarized from both the atrial and ventricular directions. The fusion beat has characteristics of both beats.

PVC s can also occur in patterns:

> **Bigeminy**- characterized by a pattern of sinus beat, PVC, sinus beat, PVC...
> **Trigeminy**- two normal beats, a PVC, two normal beats, a PVC...
> **Pairs or Salvos**- two consecutive PVC s falling together.
> PVC s falling in groups of three or more are referred to as Ventricular tachycardia.

- ♥ The frequency of PVC s increases with age as well as certain outside stimulants. They are "felt" sometimes as palpitations in the chest or neck. (Caused by a greater than normal contractile force.)
- ♥ Long runs of PVC s may cause angina or hypotension.

CAUSES

- Most drugs that are used to suppress ventricular ectopy are also known to produce it on certain occasions. Digitalis in particular will cause ventricular arrhythmias yet is very effective in controlling atrial and ventricular arrhythmias when they are related to the presence of CHF. Others include aminophylline, tricyclics, amphetamines, anesthesia induced hypoxia, and beta adrenergics such as isuprel and dopamine.
- Medical causes can include:
  - Heart failure
  - Old or acute myocardial infarctions
  - Mitral valve prolapse
  - Contusions with heart trauma
  - Catheter irritation (pacemaker leads etc.)
  - Electrolyte imbalances (hypokalemia, hypomagnesaemia)
  - Caffeine
  - Nicotine
  - Alcohol
  - Increasing age
  - Stress.
  - PVC s falling on or near the T wave can precipitate Ventricular tachycardia

TREATMENT

- Treatment varies according to the underlying cause
- In the absence of heart disease PVC s may be of no significance and require no treatment

- ♥ PVCs in asymptomatic middle-aged males may be associated with coronary artery disease and places them at an increased risk of sudden death.

- ♥ PVCs occurring with a slow ventricular rate caused by a bradycardia are best treated with atropine, or by pacing. Caution should be used though, as the increased rate will increase the myocardial oxygen demand.

- ♥ Amiodarone is the drug of choice for PVCs occurring at a fast rate.

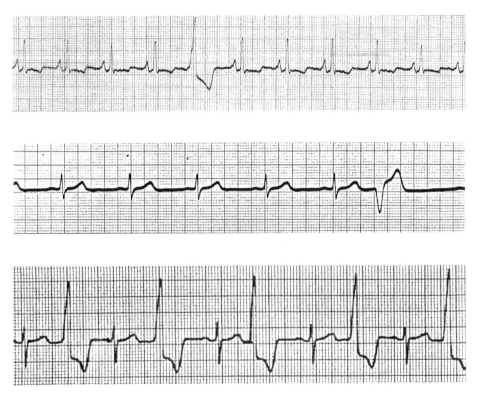

VENTRICULAR TACHYCARDIA
VT

ATRIAL   Atrial activity may be present but is usually indistinguishable due to the magnitude of the ventricular complexes. P waves will be identifiable in about 20% of the cases of VT.

    RATE

    RHYTHM

    CONTOUR

VENTRICULAR

    RATE   150-250

    RHYTHM   Regular

    CONTOUR   Abnormally wide, bizarre complexes, but uniform in contour
T waves opposite deflection of the QRS complex.

CHARACTERISTICS

- ♥ Ventricular tachycardia (VT) is probably best described as a "series of three consecutive PVC s occurring at a rate of 100 beats per minute or greater."
- ♥ The ventricular complexes occur independent of any atrial activity and are characterized by a series of wide bizarre complexes with the ST-T vector usually pointing in the opposite direction of the common QRS deflection.
- ♥ The P-R interval may be regular or irregular. If it is irregular, AV disassociation has probably occurred. The atria may be depolarized in a retrograde fashion. In this case, AV disassociation has not occurred.

Several types of VT are known:

Sustained – lasting for greater than 30 seconds

Non-sustained – short bursts of VT separated by periods of normal rhythm.

Monomorphic – appearing with a regular rate and a fixed shape on the EKG. Each beat looks the same since it is originating from the same foci.

Polymorphic- having an irregular rate and rhythm, and varying shape on the EKG. Originating from multiple foci in the ventricles.

Parasystole- A rare, usually benign independent ectopic rhythm that operates alongside the primary rhythm. From the Greek "para", meaning beside. The rhythm originates from a pacemaker in the ventricle near enough to the normal pacemaker that it is protected from invasion from outside impulses. This rhythm has two cardinal features; a variation in the coupling intervals and a common denominator in the ectopic intervals. The variation suggests the beats are from an independent mechanism.

Torsades de Pointes – "Twisting of points" characterized by a QRS contour that changes from a negative to a positive deflection and back again in a cyclic pattern with the QT interval usually greater than 0.60 sec.

Symptoms of VT depend upon the rate and the severity of the underlying heart disease. The most critical situation can be a transition to ventricular fibrillation

CAUSES

- ♥ A PVC firing on the vulnerable section of the T wave (a period of about 0.20 – 0.40 sec near the apex of the T wave) may trigger a run of VT.
- ♥ An external DC shock occurring during that vulnerable period can cause the same result. During the vulnerable period, maximum nonuniformity of the ventricular muscle is present.

- ♥ Other causes may include:
    - ♥ Ischemia (71%)
    - ♥ Myocardial irritability
    - ♥ MI
    - ♥ CAD
    - ♥ Mitral valve prolapse
    - ♥ CHF
    - ♥ Cardiomyopathy,
    - ♥ Pulmonary emboli
    - ♥ Electrolyte imbalances (potassium, magnesium)
    - ♥ Metabolic disorders (hypoxemia, acidosis)
    - ♥ Digitalis
    - ♥ Quinidine
    - ♥ Procainamide
- ♥ Runs of VT are common during reperfusion of a blocked vessel following the administration of thrombolytics

TREATMENT

- ♥ The course of treatment and the speed at which it is delivered is based upon the clinical condition of the patient.
- ♥ Unstable patients, those exhibiting symptoms such as hypotension, altered levels of consciousness, or chest discomfort, will require a more rapid approach than those presenting with stable vital signs.

- ♥ For the stable patient, medications aimed at reducing the rate and calming the ventricles, as well as correcting any electrolyte imbalances are the best choice. Those medications include: Beta-blockers, Amiodarone, Lidocaine, Procainamide, and Sotolol. Synchronized cardioversion with sedation would then follow if the medications failed to terminate the arrhythmia. The implantable cardioverter-defibrillator has become the treatment of choice for patients with recurrent life threatening VT. The device continually monitors the patient, assesses the rhythm and if indicated administers a shock to the patient to terminate the arrhythmia.
- ♥ Unstable patients should be rapidly treated with DC cardioversion.
- ♥ Pulseless patients should be treated as in ventricular fibrillation and defibrillated as soon as possible.

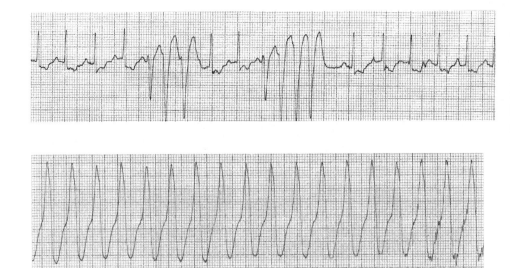

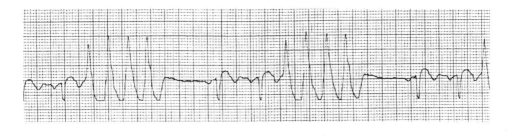

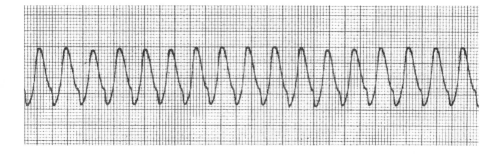

TORSADES DE POINTES

Torsades de Pointes is a syndrome rather than a rhythm description

ATRIAL

    RATE

                PRI

    RHYTHM

    CONTOUR

VENTRICULAR

    RATE   200-250

                QTI

    RHYTHM

    CONTOUR

CHARACTERISTICS

- Shifting of the QRS axis with a QT interval greater than 0.60 seconds

CAUSES

- QT prolongation leads to electrical instability that can cause cells in the ventricles to fire early
- The mechanism is unknown but evidence suggests a re-entry mechanism
- Drugs: quinidine, procainamide, amiodarone, tricyclic antidepressants,
- Electrolyte imbalances: hypokalemia, hypomagnesaemia, hypocalcaemia
- Phenothyazines
- Insecticides
- Central nervous system damages including intracranial trauma, subarachnoid hemorrhage
- Hypothyroidism

- ♥ Some congenital syndromes such as Romano Ward and Jervill & Lange-Nielson syndromes
- ♥ QT prolongation may occur with myocarditis, myocardial infarctions, and variant angina, but Torsades de Pointes is rare in these settings.

TREATMENT

- ♥ This rhythm frequently terminates itself after a short run.
- ♥ Short runs usually produce no symptoms, while longer runs may produce lightheadedness, syncope, seizures, or cardiac arrest.
- ♥ Magnesium is useful in the termination of Torsades de Pointes
- ♥ Temporary atrial or ventricular pacing has been successfully used in terminating the arrhythmia
- ♥ Prolonged episodes may require defibrillation, however, frequent repeated defibrillations make this technique less successful
- ♥ Identification and elimination of the cause of the QT prolongation should be the goal of treatment
- ♥ Distinguishing polymorphic VT (VT with the changing axis but without QT prolongation) is important since the administration of certain antiarrhythmics may increase the abnormally long QT interval and worsen the arrhythmia

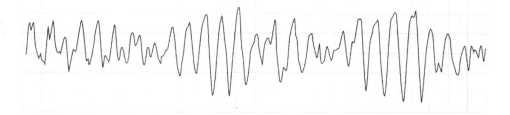

WOLFE-PARKINSON-WHITE SYNDROME

ATRIAL

    RATE   60-100
    PRI   <0.12 sec

    RHYTHM   Regular

    CONTOUR   Normal

VENTRICULAR

    RATE
    QTI   >0.12 sec

    RHYTHM

    CONTOUR   Abnormal QRS with a slurring of the R wave; called a Delta wave

CHARACTERISTICS

- Normal P wave with a P-R interval less than 0.12 seconds
- Wide QRS complex (greater than 0.12 seconds) with an initial slurring of the complex called a Delta wave
- Notched R, RS, or RSr in lead V_1
- Delta wave and the remainder of the QRS complex are negative in leads V_1 and V_2
- PSVT is the most common tachyarrhythmia seen with WPW and is usually initiated by a premature beat

CAUSES

- An accessory pathway, usually the Bundle of Kent, allows an impulse to bypass the AV junction and activate the ventricles prematurely
- The PR interval is shortened because the normal delay created by the impulse passing through the AV junction is avoided

- ♥ Hyperthyroidism
- ♥ ASD/VSD
- ♥ Transposition of the great vessels
- ♥ Tetrology of Fallot
- ♥ Most common in males
- ♥ Two thirds of the people with WPW have no associated heart disease

TREATMENT

- ♥ Sometimes patients can control some of the palpitations by holding their breath for prolonged periods of time
- ♥ Destroy the extra electrical pathway using radio frequency ablation

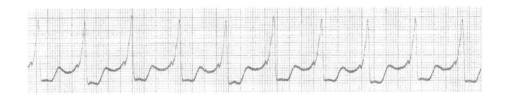

ABERRANT VENTRICULAR CONDUCTION

Aberrancy is defined as temporary abnormal ventricular conduction of supraventricular impulses, and is divided in to three forms or categories. The first form is the most common. It develops when an impulse arrives at a point in the ventricular conduction system that is still refractory and a beat is generated. When noted in the presence of atria fibrillation it often mimics ventricular tachycardia. Called Ashman's Phenomenon, it is characterized with a fast – slow- aberrant pattern.

The second form of aberration is due to anomalous conduction above the ventricles, which leads to abnormal distribution within the ventricles. This form is not dependant upon refractoriness and independent of cycle length. It usually shows a distorted ventricular complex.

The third form results from a lengthening of the ventricular cycle and may be due to spontaneous depolarization of a conducting fascicle. Only late beats are aberrant.

Clues to identifying aberrant beats:
- ♥ The presence of a preceding ectopic P wave
- ♥ Less than a full compensatory pause. Premature ventricular beats usually (but not always) have a compensatory pause that is twice the normal R –R cycle. Aberrantly conducted beats tend to have a shortened compensatory pause.
- ♥ A large majority of ectopic ventricular beats have an initial deflection different from the conducted beats, where the aberrant ones will be in the same deflection.
- ♥ In a cyclic sequence such as in atrial fibrillation, an anomalous beat ending a cycle longer than the usual cycle is more likely to be ectopic than aberrant.

These are only clues to assist in differentiating ectopic from aberrant beats. As with any situation, there are always exceptions; ventricular impulses are often conducted backward into the atria and the retrograde impulse may prematurely discharge the SA node resulting in a less than full compensatory pause, all waveforms may not be clear, and measurements may not be discernable. Don't waste time that could be spent treating the patient on deciding what name to give the rhythm.

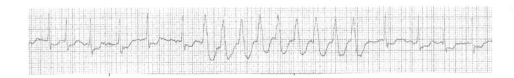

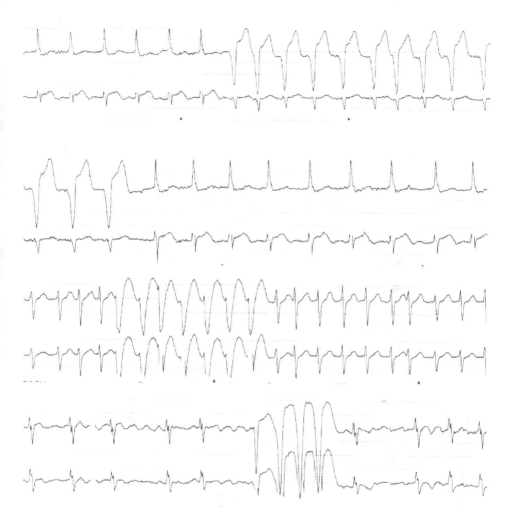

ACCELERATED IDIOVENTRICULAR RHYTHM

ATRIAL

    RATE   60-100

    RHYTHM   Regular

    CONTOUR   Normal
                           An atrial rhythm may exist independently of the ventricular rhythm

VENTRICULAR

    RATE   50 – 100 The ventricular rate usually stays within ten beats of the regular sinus rate.

    RHYTHM   May be regular or irregular

    CONTOUR   Usually wider than 0.12 seconds

CHARACTERISTICS

- ♥ Accelerated Idioventricular rhythm is characterized by a shifting of the pacemaker sites between sinus and ventricular sites with little change in the rate of the rhythm.
- ♥ The rhythm is usually transient, with episodes lasting only a few seconds to a minute. The episode commonly begins with a fusion beat.
- ♥ It is common for pacemaker sites to shift between the sinus and ventricular pacemakers in the His-Purkinje system, as both try to gain control over the slow heart.
- ♥ Onset is usually gradual and occurs when the rate of the ventricular pacemaker exceeds that of the atrial pacemaker.

- ♥ Termination is usually gradual as the rate of the sinus pacemaker increases above that of the ventricular pacemaker.
- ♥ It usually does not affect the course or prognosis of a disease.

CAUSES

- ♥ Heart disease
- ♥ Myocardial infarction
- ♥ Digitalis toxicity

TREATMENT

- ♥ Treatment is usually not necessary. As a rule, idioventricular rhythms are benign, however
- ♥ Some forms do require treatment. Those include:
- ♥ A-V disassociation resulting in the loss of AV sequential contraction with hemodynamic compromise.
- ♥ Idioventricular rhythm occurring together with more rapid forms of VT.
- ♥ Idioventricular rhythm beginning with a premature systole near the vulnerable period.
- ♥ Rapid ventricular rate which produces symptoms
- ♥ Development of ventricular fibrillation

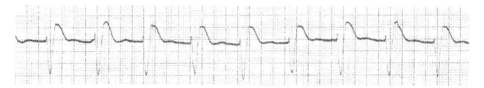

VENTRICULAR FIBRILLATION
Vf

ATRIAL

Atrial activity may be present, but is indistinguishable due to the chaotic nature of the ventricular rhythm

    RATE

    RHYTHM

    CONTOUR

VENTRICULAR

Grossly irregular. No QRS complexes are present. Rapid and chaotic rhythm

    RATE

    RHYTHM

    CONTOUR

CHARACTERISTICS

Ventricular fibrillation and ventricular flutter both represent a severe derangement of heart activity. Both rhythms usually terminate fatally in three to five minutes of onset. Immediate treatment is important.

- ♥ Ventricular flutter resembles a Sine wave with regular, large, oscillating waves.
- ♥ Ventricular fibrillation has a grossly irregular pattern varying in size and contour.
- ♥ No distinct complexes are identifiable, and differentiation between the two rhythms is of academic interest only. Both require rapid intervention of the same manner.
- ♥ Vf presents itself as unconsciousness accompanied with seizures, apnea, and eventually death if not treated. Pulse,

blood pressure, and heart sounds are undetectable, and eventually all electrical activity of the heart ceases

CAUSES

Ventricular fibrillation (Vf) occurs in a variety of situations but is usually associated with
- Coronary heart disease
- Acute MI
- Myocardial ischemia
- Advanced forms of heart block
- VT
- Electrolyte imbalances
- Hypothermia
- Electric shock
- It can occur during tissue reperfusion during thrombolytic therapy.
- It also occurs frequently as the terminal event of a variety of diseases.

TREATMENT

- Immediate defibrillation. Defibrillation within the first 30 – 60 seconds has been the most successful.
- A precordial thump may be used if the event is witnessed.

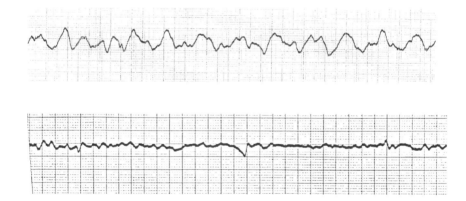

ASYSTOLE

ATRIAL

    RATE   0

    RHYTHM   None

    CONTOUR   None detectable

VENTRICULAR

    RATE   0

    RHYTHM   None

    CONTOUR   None detectable

CHARACTERISTICS
- Absence of waveforms on the monitor, confirmed in more than one lead
- No electrical activity of the heart is detected on the monitor

CAUSES
- Hypoxia
- Hypovolemia
- Acidosis
- Pulmonary embolus
- MI
- Cardiac tamponade
- Hypokalemia
- Drug overdoses; especially cocaine
- Drowning
- Electrical shock

TREATMENT
- Pacing
- Epinephrine
- Atropine

Asystole as an initial rhythm in an event is rare and return to a viable rhythm infrequent; consider the factors leading to the rhythm. Perhaps it should be considered a final rhythm, sparing the patient, family members, and caregivers the exhaustive, yet negative efforts of a prolonged resuscitation.

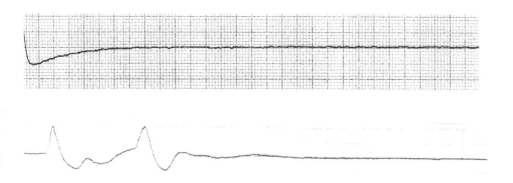

Agonal Rhythm-
- ♥ A form of asystole
- ♥ Occasional wide bizarre complexes are noted at irregular intervals
- ♥ No pulse is detected
- ♥ There is no cardiac output

Chapter Seven

Traffic Delays

Blocks

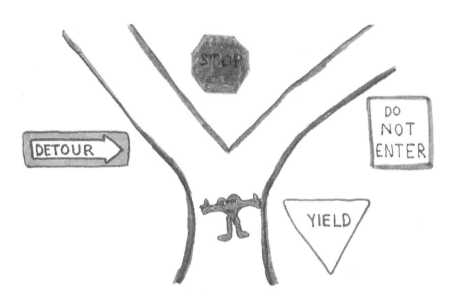

BLOCKS

A block can be defined as an abnormality of impulse conduction from the atria to the ventricles. They can be normal, physiologic, pathologic, or pharmacological in origin, and can occur at any age in either sex patient. Some go unnoticed, while others produce symptoms ranging from mild to life threatening.

Traditional classifications of blocks include: First degree; characterized by a lengthened PR interval, Second degree Mobitz I; a lengthening PR interval with a cyclic dropped beat pattern, Mobitz II; dropped beats with a usually consistent pattern, High grade AV block; a momentary absence of conduction for short (several seconds) periods of time, and Third degree; complete disassociation of the atria and ventricles.

A more precise way of describing blocks by type rather than degree is now being used. The type method of classifying blocks groups blocks according to their source of origin, but requires electrophysiology studies to determine, as the changes that occur cannot be visualized on the surface EKG.

Type I AV block occurs in the AV node and is labeled Supra-Hisian (above the bundle of His). This transient AH prolongation usually occurs during an acute MI and is often caused by ischemia. The AH interval makes up most of the PR interval on the surface EKG. This transition normally occurs over several days following the MI, and has a good prognosis.

Type II AV Block occurs in the bundle branches or fascicles (infra-Hisian) below the AV node and offers a worse prognosis than Type I. In the EP study the HV (His-Ventricular) interval represents the time interval from His bundle depolarization until the beginning of ventricular depolarization. This interval is usually short and could double without showing a noticeable first degree AV block on the surface EKG. HV prolongation during the acute MI is usually caused by necrosis and requires permanent pacemaker implantation. It is possible for this block to progress into a third degree heart block, or to a point of no escape rhythm at all with ventricular standstill. Since this block occurs below the AV junction, junctional escape impulses will be blocked and the only escape rhythm may be an idioventricular rhythm. The idioventricular rhythm will not respond to atropine, and if treated with Isuprel, may change to ventricular tachycardia. Suppression of the ventricular tachycardia may lead to asystole. The onset of complete heart block is usually sudden and without warning.

Second degree AV nodal block is diagnosed when the **entire** rhythm strip shows every other P wave conducted. Since the strip doesn't show two **consecutive** conducted P waves, PR prolongation cannot be proven therefore it is not possible to distinguish between Second degree Mobitz I and II.

High degree AV block results in a series of dropped QRS complexes – ventricular standstill. High degree AV block, when seen with Type I (supra Hisian) is usually a benign phenomenon, which may be vasovagal reactions. Vagal stimulation affects both SA and AV node conduction. When High degree AV block occurs with a Type II (infra Hisian), it can be extremely dangerous, but reverses after the vagal event has passed.

Complete Heart Block/Third Degree Block is considered one of the three forms of AV disassociation. No sinus impulses are passed to the ventricles. This can be transient lasting two to four days or may be permanent. Cardiac output can decrease leading to the development of angina or CHF.

Since the type method of defining blocks requires electro-physiology studies, only examples and definitions of the degree method of defining blocks will be discussed here.

Learning something always seems easier when you have a "system." Here is a little story that helped me to remember the degrees of blocks; it tells of four cheating husbands. Think of the husband as the P wave and the wife as the QRS complex. The PR interval represents the time each evening the husband stays out. Mr. First degree AV block was faithful; he just came home a little late each night, but always came home. Mr. Second Degree Mobitz I was a little less reliable. He came home on time the first night, stayed out a little later the next night, even later the next, and the next night failed to come home at all. Feeling bad about what he had done, he was on time the next night, but then the pattern resumed. Mr.

Second Degree Mobitz II was a little more predictable. He came home one night and then didn't come home at all the second. The next night he was on time and then once again, failed to come home. This pattern occurred over and over. Mr. Third Degree had no communication at all with his wife. He did as he pleased and she did the same, never communicating with each other.

FIRST DEGREE AV BLOCK

ATRIAL

    RATE   60-100
    PRI   > 0.20 Sec

    RHYTHM   Regular

    CONTOUR   Normal

VENTRICULAR

    RATE   60-100
    QTI   Normal

    RHYTHM   Regular

    CONTOUR   Normal

CHARACTERISTICS

- ♥ First-degree block is a conduction delay rather than a block, which occurs at the level of the AV node or Bundle of His. It produces no symptoms, but rather can be a symptom itself.
- ♥ Its only defining characteristic is the prolonged PR interval of greater than 0.20 seconds.
- ♥ All impulses are carried through to the ventricles.
- ♥ It is usually benign and rarely advances to a complete heart block.

CAUSES

- First degree AV block may appear in healthy persons without cause.
- Drugs (digitalis, procainamide, propanolol),
- Rheumatic fever
- Vagal stimulation
- Potassium imbalances
- Inferior wall MI
- Ischemia
- Infection
- A diseased AV node
- High vagal tone

TREATMENT

- Usually no treatment is required except to treat the underlying cause.
- Exercise, and medications such as atropine, isoproterenol, and steroids are known to decrease the PR interval.
- If the heart rate is slow atropine may be used to treat the bradycardia.

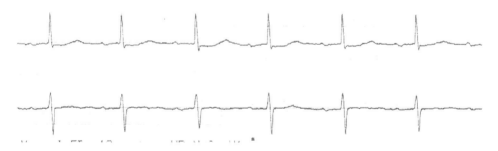

SECOND DEGREE BLOCK
MOBITZ TYPE I
WENCKEBACH

ATRIAL

    RATE   60-100
                   PRI   Progressively lengthening

    RHYTHM Regular with consistent P-P intervals

    CONTOUR Normal

VENTRICULAR

    RATE   Less than the atrial rate
                   QTI Normal

    RHYTHM Irregular, with progressively shortening R-R interval until a P wave occurs without a QRS complex

    CONTOUR Normal, as the block occurs above the Purkinje fibers

CHARACTERISTICS

- ♥ Mobitz I is characterized by the failure of certain atrial impulses to conduct when physiologic interference would not be expected-sometimes defined as periodic failure of AV conduction.
- ♥ The blockage may occur at regular (typical pattern) or irregular intervals (atypical pattern), and may be preceded by a fixed or lengthening PR interval.
- ♥ It is most commonly characterized by the lengthening PR interval until eventually a complex appears dropped.
- ♥ The R-R interval encompassing the dropped beat measures less than twice the shortest R-R interval.

- ♥ Mobitz Type I occurs most commonly in the AV junction but may also occur high in the Bundle of His.
- ♥ It is often a transient occurrence, which is 6-9% more prevalent during sleep and in athletic individuals, suggesting that vagal tone is a contributing factor.

CAUSES

- ♥ Inferior wall MI
- ♥ Digitalis or quinidine toxicity
- ♥ Vagal stimulation
- ♥ Electrolyte imbalances
- ♥ Arteriosclerotic heart disease
- ♥ Post heart surgery

TREATMENT

- ♥ Treatment is seldom necessary; find and treat the underlying cause.
- ♥ Symptomatic bradycardias may be treated with atropine and temporary pacing.

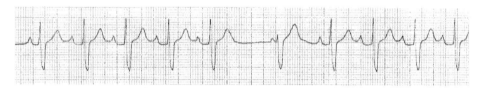

Atrial tachycardia with Wenckebach

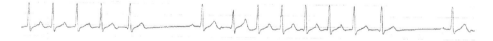

SECOND DEGREE BLOCK
MOBITZ II

ATRIAL

    RATE   60-100
                          PRI Normal or prolonged but **consistent** 2:1, 3:1, etc.

    RHYTHM   Regular

    CONTOUR Normal

VENTRICULAR

    RATE   Slow. One third to one half of the normal rate

                          QTI Normal

    RHYTHM   Usually regular

    CONTOUR Normal to slightly widened

CHARACTERISTICS

- Intermittent QRS complexes are absent without a lengthening PR interval as seen in Mobitz Type I block.
- The P waves that are conducted have a consistent PR interval, thus making the ventricular rhythm more regular.
- The P-P interval containing the non-conducted P wave equals two P-P intervals.
- This type block almost always occurs in the His-Purkinje system. Mobitz II block has several P waves for each complex (2:1, 3:1, 4:1, etc.)
- Two types are known: consistent – which occurs at regular intervals, and periodic – which occurs with irregular conduction patterns.

CAUSES

- Excessive vagal stimulation
- Drugs such as: quinidine, procainamide, potassium and Verapamil (it is usually not caused by digoxin toxicity)
- Rheumatic fever
- Chronic ischemic heart disease
- Anterior wall MI
- Hyperthyroidism
- Atrial septal defect
- Cardiac surgeries
- Hypoxia from any cause including anesthesia, and pulmonary embolism may produce significant degrees of AV block.

TREATMENT

- Mobitz II is more likely to deteriorate without warning into a greater degree of block than Mobitz I, so increasing the ventricular rate is important.
- Epinephrine, Atropine and temporary pacing are used to increase the rate until permanent pacing is available.

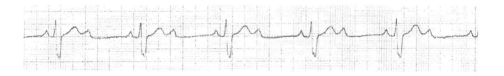

THIRD DEGREE HEART BLOCK
COMPLETE HEART BLOCK

ATRIAL

    RATE   60-100
    PRI   None

    RHYTHM   Regular. P-P intervals remain constant

    CONTOUR   Normal

VENTRICULAR

    RATE   20-40
    QTI   Normal to prolonged

    RHYTHM   Regular. R-R intervals remain constant

    CONTOUR   Normal to widened depending upon the ventricular pacemaker site

CHARACTERISTICS

- None of the impulses generated in the atria are passed through to the ventricles.
- Atrial and ventricular rhythms occur independent of each other.
- The QRS complexes will appear normal if the ventricular beat originates high in the AV junction, above the bifurcation of the AV bundle, and no bundle branch block is present, but will be wide and bizarre if the pacemaker site is in the bundle of His, or is of an Idioventricular mechanism. Keep in mind though, that distinguishing between the AV junctional pacemaker with a bundle branch block and that of an idioventricular mechanism is often impossible and will have no importance to the treatment of the rhythm.

CAUSES

- Since the ventricular rate is unusually slow more than one ventricular pacemaker may be operating simultaneously or in sequence with each other in an effort to increase the heart rate.
- Drug toxicity (digitalis)
- Degenerative heart disease producing partial to complete anatomic or electrical disruption in the AV junction, bundle of His, and Purkinje fibers; caused by fibrosis of the conduction system
- Coronary artery disease
- Myocarditis
- Inferior and anterior wall infarctions
- Age
- As a secondary effect from cardiac surgery
- Cardiomyopathy
- Less common causes include: electrolyte imbalances, endocarditis, and tumors.
- Complete heart block is rarely congenital.

TREATMENT

- Treatment is based upon both the cause and the symptoms.
- If the cause is reversible and the patient is asymptomatic then no treatment is needed other than monitoring for a deterioration of his condition.
- Complete heart block in the setting of an acute MI may require temporary transvenous pacing.
- Chronic Third degree block usually requires the insertion of a permanent pacemaker.
- Atropine would be ineffective in the treatment of complete heart block as it only increases the atrial pacemaker.

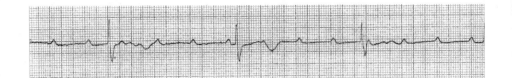

Degree	Impulses Conducted	Rhythm	PR Interval
First degree	All, but with delay	Regular	>0.20 sec consistently
Second degree Mobitz I	Some	Irregular	Lengthening Cyclic
Second degree Mobitz II	Some	Regular or irregular	Consistent for those conducted
Third degree	None	Two independent, but regular rhythms	No relationship to QRS

BUNDLE BRANCH BLOCKS

A bundle branch block is defined as a condition occurring in the bundle of His, in which impulses are blocked to one of the branches, allowing one of the ventricles to beat slightly before the other. The classic indicators are a QRS complex wider than 0.12 sec and the classic R R'. Right bundle branch blocks are seen in leads V_1 and V_2, and left bundle branch blocks are seen in V_5 and V_6.

Right Bundle Branch Block
- QRS > 0.12 seconds
- RSR' in V1 and V2 and a
- Broad S wave in leads I, V_5 and V_6
- Causes: congenital heart disease, atrial septal defect, cardiac surgery
- Prevalence: present in 0.1-0.3% of the population, occurs more frequently in males that women, and it's prevalence increases with age.
- Clinical presentation: The onset is asymptomatic, but occurs in association with pulmonary embolism, myocardial infarction, and significant coronary artery disease.

Left Bundle Branch Block
- QRS >0.12 seconds
- R in V5 and V6 and
- No Q wave in I, aVL, V_5 and V_6
- Causes: Coronary artery disease, hypertension, aortic valve disease, and cardiomyopathy.

- ♥ Prevalence: present is 0.02 – 0.3% of the population, occurs more frequently in males than females, and increases with age.

Hemiblocks are best described as an incomplete bundle branch block. The right side of the bundle branches has only one fascicle or branch, while the left has two; anterior and posterior. If conduction is delayed in only one part of the left bundle, the QRS complex will be less than 0.12 seconds.

Chapter Eight

Pacemakers

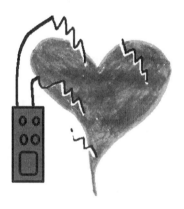

PACEMAKERS

A pacemaker is a man-made device that is used to electrically stimulate the heart muscle to contract. Pacemakers may be used to correct a variety arrhythmias including: bradycardias, tachycardias, AV blocks, and sick sinus syndrome. Currently available types of pacemakers include permanently implanted devices, temporary epicardial pacemakers and temporary external devices. A special type of pacemaker, called an Implantable Cardioverter-Defibrillator (ICD) is used to treat life threatening ventricular arrhythmias such as ventricular tachycardia. The device recognizes the arrhythmia and delivers a shock to convert the rhythm back to a normal one.

Pacemakers consist of two basic parts, the pulse generator and the lead. The pulse generator consists of the battery and electronic circuitry needed to assess and respond to the programmed needs of the patient. The pacemaker may be permanently implanted or a temporary external device used to stabilize an urgent situation.

In a permanently implanted pacemaker, the pulse generator is a small, lightweight device about the size and weight of a few stacked coins, which contains in a sealed compartment, the electronic circuitry and a battery. The circuitry is computer programmable, which allows for evaluation of the pacemaker's activity and battery life, as well as allowing the physician to change the pacemakers operation to suite the patients needs. Permanent pacemakers are indicated for chronic conditions such as symptomatic bradycardias and tachycardias, as well as heart block and recurrent life threatening arrhythmias.

Temporary pacemakers are external devices, used for short periods of time to stabilize a patient until his condition improves or a permanent pacemaker can be implanted. They are used for conditions such as hypotension and rapid arrhythmias following cardiac surgery. The device is much larger than the permanent pacemaker and has adjustable programming controls located on the unit. It remains at the bedside and limits patient mobility considerably. Temporarily implanted leads exit the patient's body and connect to the pacemaker. Temporary pacemakers use a standard household battery, which usually lasts around three to five days.

Three types of temporary pacemakers are widely used; epicardial, transvenous and external.
Epicardial electrodes are placed onto the surface of the heart during cardiac surgery and the lead wires exit through the skin just under the ribcage. The pacing leads isolated to prevent static electricity from accidentally delivering an unwanted shock, but can be quickly connected to a temporary pacemaker when needed. The end attached to the heart is shaped like a button and pulls apart into a spiral to allow easy removal simply by pulling the lead from the chest wall. Epicardial pacing allows the patient mobility during the recuperation phase.

Transvenous leads are placed through a catheter inserted into the jugular, subclavian or femoral vein, and passed into the chambers of the heart.

Trans-thoracic or external pacing can be initiated quickly, but is the least effective and most uncomfortable for the patient. Large electrodes are placed on the patient's chest and back and a shock is applied. The current must travel through the chest cavity to reach the heart muscle, so larger amounts of current are needed. If the patient is conscious, the shock may be quite uncomfortable. Good skin contact is essential and since the external electrodes are usually placed during emergency situations, skin preparation is usually minimal, movement of the patient's body is excessive, the conducting gel ends up where the adhesive of the pads should be, so they don't adhere well, and poor contact occurs. (This should not stop one form using trans-thoracic pacing! It works and saves lives!)

The leads vary according to the type of pacemaker used: permanent versus temporary. Permanent pacemakers use implanted leads that remain inside the patient's body. Temporary pacing leads are just that - temporary. They are either attached to the surface of the heart during surgery, placed into the chambers of the heart via a catheter inserted through a vein, or are attached to the external chest wall.

Each lead has small electrodes on it which function as "contact points," allowing the conduction of the electrical signal. The leads also function to carry information back to the pacemaker. A unipolar lead has one electrode, while the bipolar has two. In a unipolar lead, the electrode functions as the negative pole and the pacemakers' metal case acts as the positive pole to complete the electrical circuit. Unipolar leads are simpler to implant, but are more susceptible to intrinsic electrical activity. Bipolar leads have two electrodes. Current flows form the generator to the negative electrode at the end of the lead and returns back through the positive pole electrode to complete the circuit. Unipolar leads are less susceptible to outside interference such as skeletal muscle movement or magnetic fields, but are more difficult to implant. Lead selection varies according to the type of pacing required. For single chamber pacing, the electrode is placed n the desired chamber, either the atrium or the ventricle. For AV sequential pacing, an electrode is place in both right chambers of the heart.

Pacemaker spikes are very distinct on the EKG; in fact, some EKG displays even highlight the spike in a different color than the complex appears. The spike occurs when the pacemaker fires an electrical impulse to the heart muscle. The type of pacing determines where the spike will occur. If the patient is atrially paced the spike will be followed by a P wave and the remainder of the normal heart complex. If the ventricles are paced, the spike is followed by a QRS complex and a T wave. If the patient is AV paced, meaning paced in both the atria and ventricle, a first spike will be followed be a P wave, and after a predetermined time period, a second spike will be followed by a QRS complex and T wave. Paced complexes are electrically stimulated and usually look different from the patient's normal complex. Ventricular complexes look similar to a PVC, in fact they are an electrically induced PVC. Pacemakers are programmable to a wide variety of patient needs; so many combinations of pacing are possible. Since this book is intended as a basic or beginners guide, this is only a brief introduction and only common pacemaker rhythm examples are given.

Atrial Pacing

The pacemaker fires the atrial electrode stimulating the formation of a P wave. Note the normal appearance of the QRS complex and T wave.

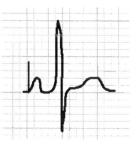

Ventricular Pacing

The pacemaker fires the ventricular electrode at a preset time after the sinus node discharges if no QRS complex is detected. Note the wide bizarre appearance of the QRS complex.

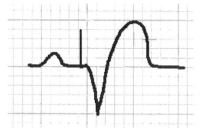

Atrial and Ventricular Pacing

The pacemaker fires the atrial electrode resulting in a P wave. If after a preset time interval no QRS complex is detected, the pacemaker fires the ventricular lead producing a QRS complex.

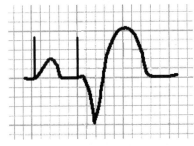

Pacemaker Classifications and Codes

Pacemakers are classified according to how they stimulate the heart. Asynchronous or fixed rate pacemakers fire at a preset heart rate regardless of the hearts own activity. These pacemakers are rarely used. Synchronous or demand pacemakers sense the heart activity and pace only when needed.

A three or five letter coding system is used to describe the pacemaker's capabilities.

First Letter Chamber Paced	Second Letter Chamber Sensed	Third Letter Response to intrinsic activity	Fourth Letter Programm-ability functions	Fifth Letter Tachy-arrhythmia functions
A Atrium	A Atrium	I Inhibits – won't fire if activity is sensed	P Basic functions programmable	P Override Pacing
V Ventricle	V Ventricle	T Triggered	M Multiprogramm-able	S Shock (ICD function)
D Dual	D Dual	D Dual	C Communicating – stores information which can be retrieved	D Dual
O None	O None	O None	R Rate modulation – adjusts rate to patient needs	O None
S Single	S Single		O None	

148

Common Pacemaker Codes

AAI – Atrial demand pacemaker. This is a single chamber pacemaker which paces and senses in the atria only. Used in patients with sinus bradycardias.

VVI – Ventricular demand pacemaker. This is a single chamber pacemaker which paces and senses in the ventricles only. It is used in patients with complete heart block.

DVI – AV sequential pacemaker. This is a dual chamber pacemaker sensing and inhibiting only in the ventricles. This type pacemaker is helpful to patients with AV block or Sick Sinus Syndrome, as it provides synchronization of the atria and ventricles therefore improving cardiac output. It isn't helpful in atrial fibrillation, as it cannot capture the atria, and the sensing of the fibrillation may cause it to fire or not fire inappropriately.

DDD – A "Universal Pacemaker." This pacemaker is used with AV block. It has many advantages including programmability and the ability to change modes automatically. Its versatility also makes it more difficult to troubleshoot. The DDD pacemaker is set with at rate range, rather than a single rate, allowing it to sense and respond atrial activity and maintain a normal AV synchronization.

Troubleshooting

A malfunctioning pacemaker can lead to problems including arrhythmias, hypotension, and syncope. Two of the most common problems are failure to capture and failure to sense.

Failure to capture is easy to spot on the EKG – pacer spikes are present but without a complex. The pacemaker senses the need and fires, but the impulse is not relayed to the tissue to cause a contraction. Causes include low output of the pacemaker due to a discharged battery, a cracked or broken lead wire, or a displaced lead, electrolyte imbalance, and acidosis.

Pacemaker spikes appearing in inappropriate places on the EKG indicate failure to sense. Spikes may be seen along with complexes generated by the hearts own intrinsic activity. This is dangerous since a misfired impulse during a vulnerable period (on the latter half of the T wave) can start a lethal rhythm such as Ventricular tachycardia. This can sometimes be corrected on temporary pacemakers by adjusting the sensitivity to a lower milliamp setting. Other causes include broken or dislodged leads, electrolyte imbalances, fibrosis at the lead electrode, and low batteries. Over sensing presents a similar problem, except it is caused by the pacemaker interpreting interference such as muscle movement as heart activity, and may cause the pacemaker to not fire when it is actually needed.

Atrial pacing

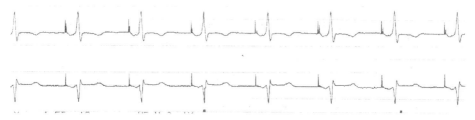

Ventricular Pacing

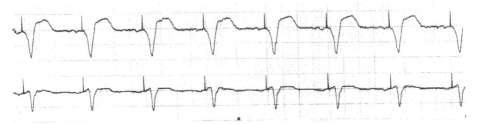

AV Sequential Pacing

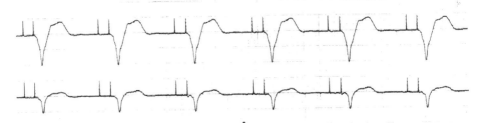

Failure to capture

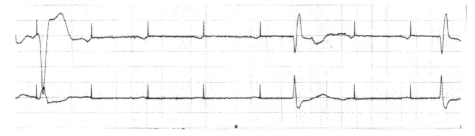

Failure to sense

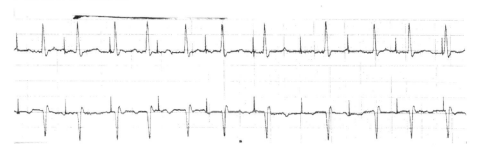

Chapter Nine

Odds and Ends...Evens and Middles

Ischemia and Infarction

Ischemia, an insufficient blood supply to the tissue, to meet the metabolic demands of the myocardium, may present with symptoms of crushing chest pain to no physical symptoms at all. Ischemia can begin within 30 seconds of the interruption of blood flow to the tissues, and angina within a few minutes of that interruption. Infarction (death of the tissue) can take 30 minutes or longer to occur.

The most often affected area of the EKG is the ST segment; with ischemia causing a depression and infarction causing an elevation of that segment from the isolectric line. By knowing which section of the heart is represented by a particular lead on the EKG, one can determine the involved area of the heart.

Non-pathologic J-point elevation can sometimes be mistaken for ST elevation. This is identified by an elevation of the terminal portion of the QRS complex which dips back toward the baseline before rising to the ST segment. In pathologic ST elevation there is no terminal portion dip back to the baseline.

After an infarction has occurred the T wave will invert and, within weeks, a Q wave may develop.

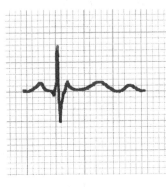 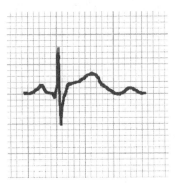

J Point Elevation   **ST Segment Elevation**

EKG Changes During the Evolution of an Infarction

Tissue deprived of oxygen dies within a short time. This is called infarction. Infarcted tissue is electrically silent. Since it does not conduct or respond to electrical stimuli, the impulses must now follow a different pathway to reach their destination. These different pathways result in alterations of the EKG waveforms. By knowing where each portion of the heart is represented on the EKG, we can identify the area of the infarct, and by knowing when these characteristic changes occur, the age of the infarct can be estimated.

Within minutes of the occlusion of the artery, J point elevation as well as ST elevation occurs in the leads facing the damaged area. This is labeled the hyperacute phase. T waves are usually tall and upright in this phase.

The period starting hours to days after onset (depending on the extent of the injury) is considered the fully evolved phase. During this period, deep T wave inversion occurs and pathologic Q waves begin to develop.

The resolution phase changes appear within a few weeks of the infarction. The ST segment returns to baseline and the T wave becomes shallow and eventually returns to normal. The Q waves, if developed, will remain permanently.

Not all infarctions produce Q waves! Full thickness damage– that is damage to all the layers of the myocardium, called a transmural infarction, usually produces Q waves, while partial thickness - called a subendocardial infarction usually does not produce a Q wave.

Axis Determination

The axis is a numerical representation of the general direction of the electrical current of the heart muscle. Axis is defined and the sum of vectors, while a vector is defined as the quantity of electrical force having a known magnitude and direction. Now that all the technical stuff is out of the way, we know that electricity traveling toward a positive electrode will produce a positively deflected complex, and traveling away from it will result in a negative complex. A current traveling perpendicular to an electrode will not produce a deflection and is therefore labeled as isolectric.

We use the six frontal leads to determine an electrical axis: leads I, II, III, aVR, aVL, and aVF.

Leads I, II, and III form the sides of an equilateral triangle, known an Einthoven's Triangle that is superimposed over the body to illustrate the limb leads. The augmented leads aVR, aVL, and aVF bisect the leads of the triangle.

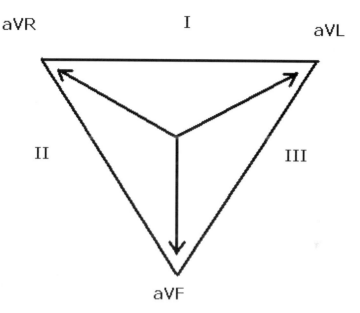

The axis is the sum of these vectors to produce a single electrical vector.

In the normal heart, this sum would be pointing down and to the left--the same general direction the impulse travels through the heart (from the top right-the SA node in the right atrium downward to the ventricles).

Two Lead Method

Using Leads I and aVF

Two leads, I and aVF, can be used to determine a general axis. Look at the QRS complex in each lead and determine if it is positive or negative. Follow the simple chart to determine the axis.

I	aVF	Axis / Deviation	Can be normal in:
↑	↑	30 – 90 ° Normal axis	
↓	↑	<30° Right axis deviation	Young thin people
↓	↓	>90° Left axis deviation	Ascites, abdominal tumors, pregnancy and obesity

Using Leads I and II

If **both** leads I and II have upright QRS complexes, the axis is **normal.**

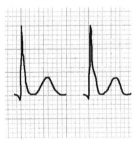

If lead I is upright and lead II is negative, **left axis deviation (LAD)** is present. This is the most common axis deviation.

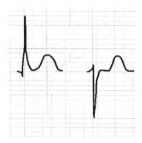

If both lead I and lead II are negatively deflected, **extreme axis deviation** is present.

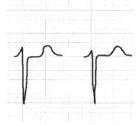

If lead I is negative (with an upright P wave), and lead II is upright, **right axis deviation (RAD)** is present.

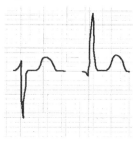

If **both** the P wave and the QRS complex are **negative** in lead I, the arm leads are **reversed.**

Perpendicular Rule

Using the frontal leads, the mean QRS vector is assumed to be perpendicular to the axis of the lead with the most equiphasic complex. The lead perpendicular to the most equiphasic QRS complex indicates the axis. The numerical value of the axis is determined by following the perpendicular lead toward the pole that is in the preselected quadrant.

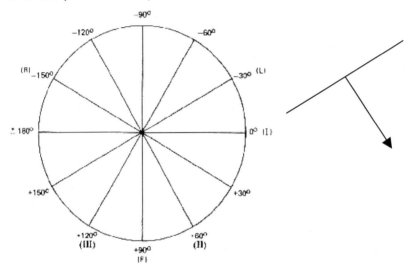

In the example above, lead aVL has the most equiphasic complex. Perpendicular to lead aVL is +60 degrees. One can assume the axis to be normal.

Predominant Polarity Method

Using leads I and aVF, one can determine the general axis by a more or less process of elimination. If the QRS in lead I is predominantly positive the axis must be in the right half of the diagram.

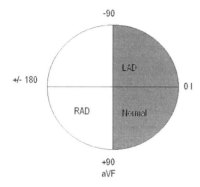

If the QRS in lead aVF is predominantly positive, then the axis must be in the bottom half of the diagram. The overlapping quadrant of the diagram indicates the axis.

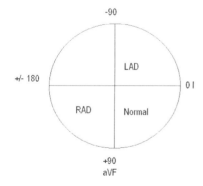

To narrow the results even further, find one of the frontal leads that is predominantly negative. The negative end of the arrow of the diagram will be in the sector of the diagram representing the axis.

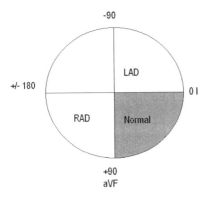

Quadrant Method

Note the deflection of the QRS complex in lead I and aVF and plot them on the chart below.

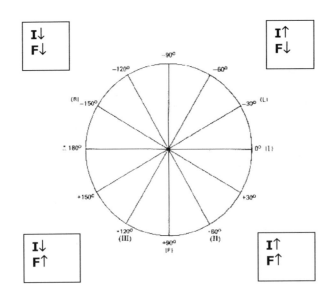

Now find the complex with the most equiphasic QRS complex, make a right angle from that lead into the quadrant indicated in the first step, and read the axis on the graph. As a confirmation, the closest identified complex should have the tallest R wave.

ATRIAL HYPERTROPHY

Thickened muscle mass in the atria increases the distance an impulse must travel, and current flow is increased in the areas of hypertrophy. This is often secondary to coronary artery or mitral valve disease.

Leads II and V_1 are the best leads for determining atrial enlargement. V_1 lies directly over the right atrium, therefore, in a normal heart, the first half of the P wave should always deflect upward and the second half should always be downward.

	LEFT ATRIAL ENLARGEMENT P MITRALE	
II	Notched P wave greater than 0.10 seconds having an M like appearance.	
V_1	Large terminal negative component of the P wave.	
	RIGHT ATRIAL ENLARGEMENT P PULMONALE	
II	Peaked P wave larger than 2.5mm	
V_1	Large initial positive component with a smaller negative terminal component.	
	COMBINED LEFT AND RIGHT ATRIAL ENLARGEMENT	
II	May be both peaked and broad.	
V_1	Biphasic peaked and broad.	

VENTRICULAR HYPERTROPHY

Left Ventricular Hypertrophy

ANY OF THE FOLLOWING:
1. ENORMOUSLY TALL QRS COMPLEXES IN THE LEADS OVER THE LEFT VENTRICLE-I, AVL, V_4, V_5, V_6
2. R IN AVL >9MM IN FEMALES OR >11MM IN MALES
3. R IN AVL PLUS S IN V_3 >20MM IN FEMALES AND >25MM IN MALES
4. R IN AVL PLUS S IN V_3 TIMES THE QRS DURATION >1847 IN FEMALES AND >2530 IN MALES
5. S IN V_1 PLUS R IN V_5 OR V_6 >35MM
6. R IN LEAD I PLUS S IN LEAD II >25MM

CAUSES:
    SYSTEMIC HYPERTENSION
    AORTIC STENOSIS OR AORTIC REGURGITATION

Right Ventricular Hypertrophy

ANY OF THE FOLLOWING:
1. RIGHT AXIS DEVIATION >90 DEGREES
2. R IN V_1 >7MM
3. RSR' IN V_1 WITH THE QRS <0.12 SECONDS
4. S >7MM IN V_5 OR V_6

CAUSES:
    CHRONIC LUNG DISEASE
    PULMONARY HYPERTENSION
    TRICUSPID REGURGITATION
    CONGENITAL LESIONS SUCH AS TETRALOGY OF FALLOT, PULMONIC STENOSIS, ATRIO-SEPTAL DEFECT, OR VENTRAL-SEPTAL DEFECT

COMMON DRUG EFFECTS
POTASSIUM

Normal: K^+ = 3.5 – 5.0
T wave is larger than the U wave

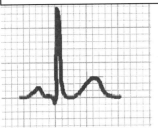

Hypokalemia: K^+ <2.6
Flat T wave with a prominent U wave

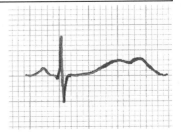

Early Hyperkalemia: K^+ 5.5 – 7.5

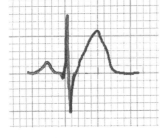

Late Hyperkalemia: K^+ >9.0

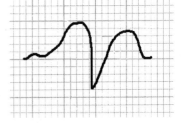

CALCIUM

Hypocalcemia Prolonged QT because of a long ST segment

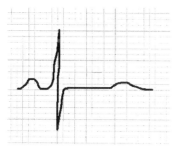

Hypercalcemia Shortened QT interval

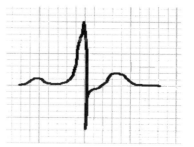

DIGITALIS

ST segment depression and sagging

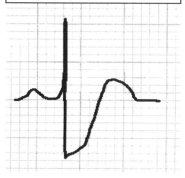

ISCHEMIA	INFARCT
ST SEGMENT DEPRESSION 0.5 MM LIMB LEADS 1 MM V LEADS	**SIGNIFICANT Q WAVES** AT LEAST 0.4 SEC WIDE AND/OR 25% THE SIZE OF THE R WAVE THAT FOLLOWS MAY BE SEEN ONLY AS POOR R WAVE PROGRESSION ACROSS THE V LEADS
INJURY	**NON Q WAVE INFARCTION**
HYPERACUTE T WAVES ST SEGMENT ELEVATION CONVEXES UPWARD 1MM LIMB LEADS, 2MM OR GREATER IN V LEADS T WAVES MAY INVERT AS ST RETURNS TO BASELINE	**PERSISTENT ST DEPRESSION** AND/OR **T WAVE INVERSION** LASTING GREATER THAN ONE WEEK CORRELATING WTH **ENZYME ELEVATION**

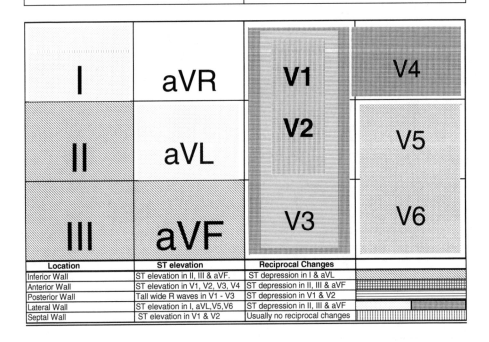

Location	ST elevation	Reciprocal Changes	
Inferior Wall	ST elevation in II, III & aVF.	ST depression in I & aVL	
Anterior Wall	ST elevation in V1, V2, V3, V4	ST depression in II, III & aVF	
Posterior Wall	Tall wide R waves in V1 - V3	ST depression in V1 & V2	
Lateral Wall	ST elevation in I, aVL,V5,V6	ST depression in II, III & aVF	
Septal Wall	ST elevation in V1 & V2	Usually no reciprocal changes	

ABERRANT VENTRICULAR CONDUCTION, 113
ACCELERATED IDIOVENTRICULAR RHYTHM, 116
ACCELERATED JUNCTIONAL RHYTHM, 95
ASYSTOLE, 121
ATRIAL FIBRILLATION, 83
ATRIAL FLUTTER, 86
ATRIAL HYPERTROPHY, 164
ATRIAL TACHYCARDIA, 79
ATRIOVENTRICULAR NODE, 15
AXIS DETERMINATION, 156
BIPOLAR LEADS, 23
BLOCKS, 125
BUNDLE OF HIS, 15
CALCULATING THE RATE, 52
COMMON DRUG EFFECTS, 166
COMPLETE HEART BLOCK, 127
COMPLETE HEART BLOCK, 134
ELECTRICAL ANATOMY OF THE HEART, 13
FIRST DEGREE AV BLOCK, 128
HIGH DEGREE AV BLOCK, 126
INTERNODAL PATHWAYS, 14
J POINT, 45
JUNCTIONAL RHYTHM, 91
JUNCTIONAL TACHYCARDIA, 95
LEAD PLACEMENT, 23
LEFT BUNDLE BRANCH BLOCK, 137
LEFT VENTRICULAR HYPERTROPHY, 165
LIMB LEADS, 23
MAT, 81
MULTIFOCAL ATRIAL TACHYCARDIA, 81
P WAVE, 39
PAC, 74
PACEMAKER CLASSIFICATIONS AND CODES, 146
PACEMAKERS, 140
PJC, 93
P-R INTERVAL, 40

PRECORDIAL LEADS, 23
PREMATURE ATRIAL CONTRACTIONS, 74
PREMATURE JUNCTIONAL CONTRACTIONS, 93
PREMATURE VENTRICULAR COMPLEXES, 99
PSVT, 63
PVC, 99
Q WAVE, 44
QRS COMPLEX, 41
QT INTERVAL, 49
RIGHT BUNDLE BRANCH BLOCK, 137
RIGHT PRECORDIAL LEADS, 24
RIGHT VENTRICULAR HYPERTROPHY, 165
SECOND DEGREE AV NODAL BLOCK, 126
SECOND DEGREE BLOCK, 130, 132
SICK SINUS SYNDROME, 72
SINUS ARREST, 68
SINUS ARRHYTHMIA, 66
SINUS BLOCK, 70
SINUS BRADYCARDIA, 59
SINUS NODE, 14
SINUS RHYTHM, 57
SINUS TACHYCARDIA, 61
ST SEGMENT, 45
SUPRAVENTRICULAR TACHYCARDIA, 63
T WAVE, 47
THIRD DEGREE BLOCK, 127
THIRD DEGREE HEART BLOCK, 134
TORSADES DE POINTES, 108
UNIPOLAR LEADS, 23
VENTRICULAR FIBRILLATION, 118
VENTRICULAR TACHYCARDIA, 103
VT, 103
WANDERING ATRIAL PACEMAKER, 77
WAP, 77
WENCKEBACH, 130
WOLFE-PARKINSON-WHITE SYNDROME, 111

ISBN 1412017106

Made in the USA